THE
JIHAD GERM

A NOVEL OF BIOTERRORISM
AND NATIONAL SECURITY

by T.N. Rivers

Pirate Island Press
Mobile, AL

www.jihadgerm.com

Library of Congress PCN 2007-936802

Printed in the United States of America

ISBN: 978-0-9799326-0-1

Chapter 1

FATHU AL-SHAMAL FACTORY

Tehran; August 2008

Tehran's morning sun illuminated the burnished bronze of the distant Fata mosque's minaret and its fine coating of gray dust. The same gray dust, sprinkled with irregular stones, covered the Fathu al-Shamal courtyard beneath the group's feet. The Iranian Imperial Guards at the electrified gate stood with their weapons at port arms as the prisoner's procession entered the small enclosure.

With tenement-dog ferocity, an aging mullah led the punishment parade, his white beard confidently resting upon the thickly padded breast of his clerical *qabaa*. Two youthful Pasdaran Revolutionary Guards followed, leading the prisoner by the leather thongs secured to his wrists.

The prisoner was young, an Iranian Shia, wearing thick glasses, a traditional, earth-toned *sherwal* with a drawstring at the waist, and a T-shirt whose calligraphy portrayed work from the poet Omar Khayyam. The prisoner's face was a pasty, pale mask of terror and shocked disbelief. The ghazi dominated the rear of the procession, with the hilt of a three-foot Iberian scimitar solidly in his right palm and the experienced, curved blade of the weapon cradled like an infant in the crook of his left arm.

The scientists and technicians stood uncomfortably, for they knew well the man who stood accused. Shahlim was twenty, a laboratory assistant who was always early for work and shared his quiet smile when asked about camera-phone pictures of his young son.

The ream of printer paper could have been in his car for reasons other than theft.

Dr. Khalid Atoomb shielded his face with his right hand as the sunlight's glint off the scimitar blade flashed into his eyes. Atoomb, thirty-two, was an Iraqi scientist who ascended to the position of research chief after working in the Republic of Iran for nearly a decade. Atoomb wore Western jeans, a floral-patterned T-shirt, and white Adidas tennis shoes. His years of education in biomedical engineering at Michigan State and in microbiology at UC–Davis fueled his desire for casual clothes ... and gave him questions about the role of the old ways in a modern world.

"For the crime of theft against the Republic of Iran," intoned the mullah, "a sacrifice is required by the law of the Qur'an. We, the Faithful, struggle in the battle with ourselves, a battle this man has lost."

The mullah nodded to the Iranian military policemen, who pushed the prisoner into a kneeling position and secured his right hand to a cylindrical block of wood in the center of the factory's courtyard.

With no further hesitation, the ghazi's scimitar stroke sliced through skin, muscle, and bone, rudely scattering four fingers in the gray dust. The severed digits grew progressively more purple and oozed drops of blood.

"Allah *Ahkbar*!" called the mullah, and the crowd dispersed, leaving Khalid Atoomb, his research assistant, Jalil, and three other loiterers in the courtyard.

"The law is clear and unmistakable," murmured Jalil, "and public punishment ... appropriate."

"I'm not so sure ...," Atoomb muttered.

"Doctor!" whispered Jalil. "Someone may hear you!"

Atoomb looked into the distance at the morning sunlight reflecting from the dust-dulled bronze of the mosque's minaret. He heard the distant screeching buses and honking taxis, but his mind remained on the severed, dust-contaminated fingers—and on the digits that remained attached to his own hands. He needed results, *now*, or even more life-threatening separations of bodily tissue could be his fate.

Atoomb turned and passed the rigid, uniformed sentry as he entered the factory's main administrative floor. He followed Jalil mechanically to the elevator, his organized mind racing as they waited for the doors to open. The pair stepped onto the worn carpeting of the elevator and entered the security code to reach the concealed laboratory three floors below the factory's administrative offices.

As the scientists entered the Liam 9 Laboratory's main salon, Jalil recaptured his position before the aged 486 computer and resumed the task of entering research data into the secure intranet.

Without speaking, Atoomb walked through the laboratory work area and entered containment Zone One, where he undressed and placed his glasses and clothing in a wall locker. Atoomb, a slight man whose receding hairline was accentuated by the long, dark hair that he combed to the rear, stood before the photoelectric trigger until the polished glass door slid open and allowed him to move forward, naked, into containment Zone Two.

In the middle containment zone, he showered, pulled

his hair into a sterile surgical cap, and then donned a one-piece plastic containment suit with hood. He plugged the suit's air hose into the Zone Two test port and inspected the suit for leaks. He pulled the suit's protective gloves onto his thin hands, taped the cuffs of the gloves for extra security, then pulled a pair of sterile surgical gloves over the bulky first layer. With confidence in his class A suit protection but gnawing fear for his future, Atoomb waited for the opening of the door into the "hot" Zone Three.

The Zone Three lab always brought a wave of pride to Dr. Atoomb. He had personally selected the expensive German centrifuges and 100-liter fermenters. He had chosen the gas chromatography equipment for the separation of proteins and developed the affinity techniques for concentrating the product. His greatest joy came from the new Micropulse gene gun, capable of firing minute fragments of DNA into a host cell without damage to the receiving cell.

His thoughts returned to the years he spent in the United States and his fond memories of Imam Siddiqi of the Sacramento mosque. When Atoomb had discussed his studies, the old man had smiled and folded his hands in supplication to Allah.

"Your work, young Faithful, is a great *barakah*, a blessing from Allah to level the playing field between these arrogant Americans and our people," said the old religious leader. "You have the tools of Jihad—tools for a mighty holy war that will bring the Americans to their knees and help to establish the *Ummah Wahidi*, the one Islamic world."

The imam had then taken a sip of tea.

"We fight the unbelievers, until they and the Great Satan's perverted government of men are in submission to Allah's will!"

Now, it had been a long six years since Atoomb had returned to his father's home in Mosul, Iraq, after completing his education in the United States. After Atoomb had spent three days in the dusty place with more sheep than humans, two men wearing dark business suits visited him. The young government men both wore their hair in short, Western cuts and spoke without traces of a smile.

"You are needed for the greater good of your people," the young official quietly pointed out. He seemed to be the leader and carried a briefcase secured to his wrist by a thin, stainless steel wire.

The official spoke in general terms of a research organization with work of great importance for the progression of Islam. The young man possessed power and confidence, tools that Atoomb had desired since his early childhood among the sheep. The newly Ph.D'ed Khalid Atoomb agreed to accompany the messengers the following morning, and later that day, he began to pack his jeans and books into a pair of battered suitcases. It was hours after the train departed Mosul that Atoomb learned that the trio's destination was Iran.

Atoomb spent four long years deep in Iran at the Hamadan laboratory, sharing his knowledge of microbial genetics and developing new capacities to manipulate the characteristics of his organisms. He moved to Tehran to develop the new laboratory beneath the Fathu-al Shamal factory and worked sixteen-hour days assembling the twenty-first-century equipment his delicate work required.

Two very long years flew by in preparation for the project, and Atoomb was terrified that the results would not come quickly enough or be impressive enough. There was not only the investment of his time; there was the investment of an unbelievable amount of money from sources unknown to him. He had solved the problems of the gene expression and worked through more than sixty failed attempts before any successful production could be verified.

If they will just ... give me the time! screamed the scientist's organized mind.

The intercom system on the Zone Three laboratory wall crackled into life.

"Doctor Atoomb!" called Jalil from the main salon. "You have been summoned to see General Madmudiyeh. His office said *immediately*!"

Fear reached deep into Atoomb's chest and squeezed his heart into a tiny lump of malleable clay.

Atoomb emptied the contents of the beaker into a reclamation sink, where the experimental fluids underwent the automatic addition of concentrated bleach, followed by exposure to high-dose radiation to prevent the product's entry into the sewer system.

Atoomb briefly stood before the inner lab's photoelectric eye and exited into lab Zone Two when the thick glass door slid open. He stood beneath the automatic showers and heard the reclamation pumps cycle the runoff water for processing. Atoomb peeled off the containment suit and dropped it into a chute for its radiation and gas sterilization. He removed the gloves last and tossed them into a hazard chute for destruction.

Atoomb entered lab Zone One, repeated his shower, and quickly dressed. He reviewed his carefully trimmed beard and his receding hairline in the locker room mirror. New wrinkles of worry and sleeplessness creased the corners of his eyes. He put on his glasses and worn lab coat and entered the laboratory's main salon, planning to tie his tennis shoes during the elevator's transit.

Jalil looked up expectantly from his work, his eyes alight with admiration for his mentor and excitement due to the important work they shared.

"Does the product concentration improve, Doctor?" asked the dedicated understudy.

"Yes, Jalil," Atoomb answered.

You see only the counselors' praise for our research success, he thought, *not the slitting of our bellies if we fail!*

With hands trembling, Atoomb walked from the main salon into the hallway beyond, followed by a trotting Jalil. Atoomb repeatedly punched an elevator "Up" button, as though the machine could sense his urgency.

"At least the elevator was made in this century," Atoomb mumbled as the doors opened and he stepped inside, trailed by his assistant. The machinery hummed as the compartment rose to the ground level of the factory.

The elevator doors opened to reveal the first-floor hallway into the Fathu al-Shamal factory's shabbily carpeted administration area. The laboratory buried beneath the factory was populated by white coats, computers, and quiet, thoughtful men, but it reported to the administrative area's military chain of command. The men who prowled the administrative halls understood power—and used punishment as just another military tactic.

Atoomb could see at the distant door an Iranian Army guard, grim faced and cradling the polished stock of his AKS-74U rifle. The scientist quickly traversed the hallway and stopped before General Madmudiyeh's door. Jalil waited outside of the office, in the unsmiling guard's line of vision. Atoomb's fear grew into terror as he imagined the dark, threatening eyes of the project director. Atoomb knocked cautiously.

"Enter!" said a gravelly voice from inside.

General Madmudiyeh sat behind a desk in the stark office, a Gauloise burning in the ashtray before him. At fifty-four, the officer exuded the fatigue of too many years in service to the Republic and wore a long scar on the right side of his face as a souvenir. His dark eyes were cold and penetrating as he looked from Atoomb's face to his Western tennis shoes, which remained untied. Atoomb glanced down at the general's omnipresent side arm.

The office held a single framed picture of the Ayatollah and a computer terminal that the general had never used. A small, scuffed bookshelf held the Holy Qur'an and several manuals on military intelligence. The aging warrior offered no greeting or welcome.

"Dr. Atoomb here as you have requested, General," said the scientist quietly.

The general did not speak but only pushed an open letter into Atoomb's reach. As he read the words on the page, Atoomb felt as if the weight of the entire factory rested upon his shoulders.

"But, General ..." Atoomb said numbly. "The date is only three weeks away!"

"You have had two years, Atoomb!" thundered the general. "Two years, and over one hundred billion rials! Do you think you can just ask for more time? You fool! Neither of us has families of power; I will hang beside you! In three weeks, the Committee of Counselors will expect a full accounting of the readiness of the project. You will deliver it, or I will kill you myself!"

"Yes, General," Atoomb heard his distant voice reply. "Allah Ahkbar."

As the terrified, bespectacled scientist departed, the general spat a fragment of French tobacco into the pile of papers on his desk.

"Academic fools," he fumed. *They know nothing of the real planning, the risks—and the lives at stake if we fail.*

The Committee of Counselors in both Tehran and Damascus were politically impenetrable; however, they would quickly sacrifice an aging intelligence general with no family wealth and a quaking young scientist.

Powerful men with powerful political friends were behind the millions in Saudi and Kuwaiti oil dollars that funneled through the Al-Bukara Bank to the Brotherhood of Islamic Jihad and the Muslim Liberation Front. There were also the American religious leaders who upheld the faith in the very face of the Great Satan and controlled the U.S. mosques and conferences that added funding to the downfall of a domi-neering world power. These rich sheiks and the American religious leaders were men he could not afford to disappoint. The containers would hold much embarrassment for the Americans, and these men would relish the victory.

Atoomb, still pale and shaking, gathered Jalil from the hallway and forced himself down the hallway to the elevator. Once safely inside, Atoomb turned to his assistant with deep concern on his face.

"We must begin the animal tests immediately," he began. "We have no more time."

Khalid Atoomb could almost feel the slice of the blade across his abdomen. He wondered if a victim remained conscious to watch his own intestines spill from his body onto the floor.

Chapter 2

JEFFERSON

Philadelphia; August 2008

J efferson Medical College, the largest privately owned, state-assisted healthcare teaching institution in the nation, upheld a long tradition of caring for thousands of Philadelphia's traumatized, plus innumerable referrals for tertiary medical care from the neighboring Pennsylvania counties. The Thomas Jefferson University Hospital's history of caring for the poor and unwashed began in 1825 and continued, despite the millions in cutbacks in the state's educational budget, largely due to the contributions of patrons.

During each twenty-four-hour day, the Jefferson emergency department could expect the usual cadre of the drunk and homeless, the occasional exotic disease referral, and several of the all-drugged-up-and-no-place-to-go. The health care ills were the easy part. One could always give an antibiotic or pain medication, or even arrange admission to the hospital if the illness was serious. The hard part was that, often, the patients had no home, no family, no food, and no expectation that upon leaving the emergency department they could expect a better life.

Emergency physicians always meet the strangest people at three or four in the morning. "Rock people" crawl from beneath their hiding places in every major U.S. city during the cool, wee hours of early morning and ride, walk, or push shopping carts to the doors of emergency departments just like Jefferson's. Patients arrive in triage, undergo evaluation to determine the severity of their illness, and then wait through tedious hours for the only source of care available to them. Urgently ill patients receive immediate care, but the people who come to an ER for a rash or a toothache often spend the night in a waiting area.

This night shift at Jefferson was no different, and Dr. Ron Raines waded through the charts of falls, fractures, and childhood fevers through the early morning hours. At three a.m., the emergency department team heard from a surgical resident that the nine-year-old girl sent to surgery with pelvic fractures from a car accident died in the operating room. The mood in the department was somber as Raines pulled the next chart from a door and prepared to enter the examination room.

"Major medical ambulance, Dr. R!" called Karen Winslow, the night triage nurse. "Temp of 103 and low pressure ... going to resuscitation three!"

Karen was the most experienced nurse on the shift and held the highly important job of seeing triage patients and making hard decisions about who should receive care next.

At forty-one, Karen was a veteran of over eighteen years in the Jefferson University emergency department. She had long, dark hair and a shape a little on the heavy side. She always wore a smile, regardless the hour of the day or number of people waiting to receive care. She kept a mental tally of the beds available and always seemed to find room to put the truly sick.

Two minutes later, the Philadelphia Fire EMS crew rolled in a gurney that held a tiny grandmother who seemed even smaller since she no longer had legs. Karen directed the EMS team into resuscitation room three, where Christie Fellows, the resuscitation room's primary nurse, prepared for the arrival's care.

Karen assessed the elderly woman and glanced at the record from the nursing home, which noted fever, shaking, and chills. Christie rapidly started an intravenous line in one of the thin arms, which were stroke-ravaged and scared down into a permanently flexed position.

Raines entered the resuscitation bay and saw an ancient gnome with a stomach tube for feeding and amputation stumps where she had once had legs. Her open-mouthed stare hinted that her brain last recognized family members many years before. An old catheter bag hanging from the gurney contained the dark, cloudy urine that likely teemed with bacteria capable of moving into her ancient bloodstream.

"Better add blood cultures, Christie," added Raines. "I'd give her a liter bolus of saline and two grams of cefepime. I'll call the ICU resident."

"Cultures are already done," Christie grinned. Her pretty face and flaming-red hair made her appear flamboyant, but her southern childhood had produced a quietly confident young lady who was a very good nurse and still cared for others.

"Sorry about the little girl, Dr. R," Christie said quietly. "I don't know what else we could've done."

Raines followed Christie and stood near her outside of the treatment room's door. He shrugged and shook his head.

"Sometimes I wonder about our priorities," said the doctor,

feeling older than he looked. "We can't save the one with her entire life ahead of her and can't let go of the one who last lived twenty years ago."

"This little lady probably has a family who loves her," Christie said.

"If they really loved her and understood how she's living, they'd just let her go," responded Raines.

As Christie watched the physician begin to write the lab and antibiotics orders on the diabetes-and-stroke-ravaged grandmother's chart, Karen approached from triage and interrupted an almost peaceful moment.

"Trauma code four minutes out, Dr. Raines. Going to resuscitation room one."

"What's the story, Karen?"

"GSW to the right chest with respiratory distress and hypotension. I've already called the surgery resident."

In even less than four minutes, Philadelphia Fire's Medic 22 crew exploded through the sliding triage doors, their arrival punctuated by the screams and curses of the teenager on the stretcher. The young man's gasping mouth revealed a gold front tooth that matched a gold chain hanging from his neck. He wore large, baggy shorts that covered his thighs, but barely reached his hips. As he struggled to exhale, he sprayed a mist of blood from the small bullet hole visible in the right side of his chest.

"I got shot—*bad!*" the young victim screamed. "You gotta *fix* me!"

Karen drove a large-bore IV line into his left arm as Raines ripped open the patient's blood-soaked T-shirt. Raines pulled over a chest tube tray from a supply rack to his rear and tossed it onto a Mayo stand at the teen's right side. The physician jammed his hands into sterile gloves and splashed antiseptic solution on the young man's chest. Raines pulled lidocaine into a syringe and injected the local anesthetic into the space between the teen's ribs, just below his heaving right nipple.

He continued to scream. Raines made a two-inch incision over the right fifth rib and then pushed a large Pean clamp through muscle and into the chest cavity. When Raines spread the clamp inside the chest, a shower of blood and air exploded onto the gurney, the wall, and the physician. With the air pressure within the chest released, the young man stopped screaming, began to breathe more easily, and grew a puzzled facial expression.

"Hey, man … you got that thing inside of me?" he asked in amazement.

"Yeah, and ain't you glad?" Raines responded.

The doctor then placed a large, plastic chest tube through the incision and sutured it into place. Karen attached suction to the end of the chest tube and called for a chest x-ray—stat.

Raines stripped off the gloves and shuffled toward the call room in search of a clean set of scrubs.

When he was out of earshot, Christie called across the trauma room—"Hey, Karen... I think this Raines guy is okay."

"I hear he's had a pretty long road for a guy for his age," Karen said. "He's got a lot more experience than most of the new attending docs. He sure doesn't wait for the surgeons to get here."

Thirty-eight-year-old Dr. Ronald Edward Raines was compact and muscular, with thick, dark brows and a well-trimmed moustache. He had been born into less than elegant circumstances in El Dorado, Arkansas, but providence had given him a father who expected things of him.

Manuel Raines was a widower, a former factory worker disabled by the thunderclap-sudden rupture of a cerebral blood vessel that left him partially paralyzed on the right side and forced to shuffle along using a cane. Manuel Raines still believed that rewards followed hard work and honesty, despite his own life having proved just the opposite.

"Leave this place," he counseled Ron, "and find a way to make a difference with your life. You are young and strong and smart; don't limit your vision of what you can do."

Into the sponge-like mind of his young son, he instilled a voracious appetite for life outside of southern Arkansas and for the chance to try new things.

Young Ron Raines, however, did not know that, during his freshman year, his father had visited Truman High School to discuss his son's educational future.

"I don't want him to be stuck here with me," the elder Raines confided to the guidance counselor. "You gotta help him find a way out."

The Truman High guidance counselor summoned Ron in January of his sophomore year and provided an option to life in southern Arkansas.

"A place called Marion Military Institute in Alabama is advertising educational opportunities for motivated young men. The school combines high school with a junior college curriculum and gives a U.S. Army commission as a second lieutenant upon graduation. I called to inquire about opportunities for out-of state students and found that there is a scholarship application process for kids like you who might participate in the school's sports program. You interested in playing football and becoming an army officer?"

"Yes, sir," nodded young Raines. "I'm sure interested."

~

The Greyhound bus's diesel roar propelled its meandering through the southern Louisiana farmlands and bayous. The fat, gnarled trunks of cypress trees rose from the dark green algae-laden pools along the highway, and heavy gray beards of moss hung from the tree's upper branches in a sweeping canopy that shaded the toads and gators that lounged beneath. Snowy egrets flapped their transit into the next tree line under the watchful eyes of red-shouldered hawks, and an occasional sleepy owl awaited dusk and another night to hunt for field mice. Throughout the long bus ride across Mississippi's Interstate 20, Raines had thought only of his father's pride if he were able to don the uniform of an army officer. Perhaps it would be an accomplishment the determined old man would find befitting his son's potential.

The bus stopped in front of an open parade ground in the tiny town of Marion, Alabama, where the thin but muscular youth gathered his father's well-worn suitcase and nervously stepped into the next phase of his life. Ron Raines would have to rely on himself to produce results—or to return to Arkansas in shame.

During February, Raines learned to wear the Marion cadet uniform and suffer the hazing of the juniors and seniors without complaint. In March, spring football training began, and Raines earned his position as a linebacker for the MMI Tigers. During the next three and a half years, he worked hard. With some surprise, he found that he did well in science and history, in addition to earning his keep in sports. His mastered the rifle range, the land navigation course, and the small-unit leadership tactics expected of a new military officer.

Ron Raines's proudest moment was walking across the Marion Institute auditorium stage as his father grinned, shaking the commandant's hand, and feeling his father pin on the gold insignia of a "butter-bar" U.S. Army second lieutenant.

Raines's first military assignment, to Ft. Benning, Georgia, provided him the opportunity to "volunteer" for the Army Airborne Course. Although sensible individuals do not enjoy jumping from perfectly good airplanes, Raines found the three weeks of five-mile runs and the five awkward plunges onto Fryar drop zone another chance to prove to his father that he could do difficult things. He was selected as one of the two honor graduates of his cycle and had the silver airborne wings pounded into his chest as the "blood wings" of graduation.

"I'm not finished yet," he told one of his black-hat instructors. "'Rangers lead the way,' and I'm going to be one."

In fact, it took six months for Raines to receive his orders for Ranger training, which gave him time to prepare with long afternoon runs and twenty-mile hikes with a sixty-pound rucksack. Yet when he entered the Ranger course and completed the swamp phase, he wished it had taken six years to find a spot in the class. Rare meals and even rarer sleep during the grueling training broke men physically and mentally, but Raines remained among the one-third of the candidates who completed the course. He added the coveted left shoulder Ranger tab to his "tree-suit."

Raines moved into the strange life of a 75th Rangers platoon leader at twenty years of age. He greeted each day with a six-mile run and suffered through a twenty-mile ruck march monthly, yet he felt strong, felt that he was beginning to earn the respect of the twelve soldiers in his command. He spent his nights learning science and math through the Troy University campus located on Ft. Benning. Raines felt more than a bit surprised when he cranked out A's and B's despite his grueling daytime schedule and became a college junior after just twenty-two months.

A desert half a world away changed many of his views about his power and his ability to handle anything. Sergeant First Class Benton was his "team daddy," ten years older than Raines. As the senior enlisted man in the platoon, Benton was the one who added controlled judgment to the unbridled testosterone of the younger solders. In the opening hours of Operation Desert Storm, on an airfield near Basra, Benton took a sniper's bullet through the neck, just above the left collar of his ballistic vest. Raines applied pressure to the hemorrhaging wound and prayed as he watched the pale, sweaty face of his NCO.

"I'll be alright, LT," croaked Benton. "Just keep the boys under cover."

Raines knew that he would not be all right, and he help-
lessly watched as Benton died before the Blackhawk medevac
chopper arrived.

I should have done more, he thought as the Rangers flew back
to Ft. Benning.

He kept his decision a secret, but in late 1991, at a much
more mature twenty-two years of age, he applied to attend
medical school at the Uniformed Services University of the
Health Sciences.

USUHS, "U Shues" in casual conversation, was a long shot,
if not an impossibility, for the young lieutenant. The admissions board was even more selective than at most medical
schools, due to the massive numbers of Army, Navy, and Air
Force servicemen and women desiring a medical education
at the government's expense. If he were selected for the class,
Raines would owe the Army seven years of service for his four
years in medical school and would add another three years of
service obligation for residency training. The service Raines
would owe made staying in the Army until retirement the only
sensible option.

Young Lieutenant Raines dutifully completed the lengthy
application packet, signing a release for his undergraduate
grades, permission for the school to contact his commander,
and a contract accepting knowledge of the obligation for
years of payback service to the government. He spent most
of his application time on his personal statement, the reasons
why he desired to become a physician and what he wanted to
accomplish if given the opportunity.

Following an eventful three-month rotation to the Pana-
manian-Columbian border, that he was not free to discuss
due to the mission's classification, Raines returned to his tiny
apartment on Victory Drive near Ft. Benning's front gate. He
picked up his accumulated mail from the apartment's office
and leafed through flyers for things he didn't want and offers
for things he couldn't afford. Near the center of the stack

was a letter from the military medical school in Bethesda, Maryland.

That would be my rejection letter, thought Raines as he flipped over and then opened the thin envelope.

"LT Raines," he read, "It is the pleasure of the Admissions Committee to accept your application for the Uniformed Services University of the Health Sciences School of Medicine class matriculating in August, 1992. Enclosed is a request for personnel action to be executed by your command, points of contact for questions, and a list of required freshman texts. Welcome to the USUHS Class of 1996."

A navy commander's signature was on the letter, and Raines read it again to ensure he had not been the subject of some cruel joke. After a walk around the block to gather his thoughts, he called his father in Arkansas.

"A doctor?" the older man asked in disbelief as he shuffled back to his chair. "Do you think you can really be a doctor?"

"Just don't remind me that I shouldn't try to be one," said young Raines. "You're the one who pushed me to see beyond Arkansas. I'll go for it—and I won't quit."

It was hard for Raines to concentrate on patrols and training his soldiers during the next seven months. He did not tell anyone that he was going to medical school until he departed for Maryland in July.

The four years of professional school flew by; gross anatomy, physiology, and pharmacology burned the months away. Raines traveled to rotations in obstetrics at Ft. Bragg and emergency medicine at Ft. Hood. His days were exciting, but more importantly, he felt that each thing he learned added tools to his toolkit. His father no longer expressed disbelief at the things Raines learned and did not seem surprised when he walked across the Bethesda stage in 1996 to receive his M.D. degree and Army captain's bars.

His specialty was emergency medicine, and Raines slogged through three long years of night shifts and critical care in the

EM residency program at Ft. Lewis, Washington. He enjoyed bone-deep fatigue, punctuated by noon conferences to discuss the care of patients while surrounded by more senior faculty physicians who always seemed well rested. He did well on his College of Emergency Physicians in-service training exams and received his orders for his next duty station three months before his residency graduation in 1999.

The army had plans for a young captain with seven years of obligated service, and an Airborne and Ranger-qualified physician was a rarity. Raines was assigned as the battalion surgeon for the First Battalion of the Fifth Special Forces Group (Airborne). He would be providing care for Ft. Bragg Green Beret soldiers and directing the activities of 18-Delta Special Forces medics. Each SF Group covered a geographic area of specialization, and the Fifth Group's language and cultural training was geared toward activities in Asia and the Middle East.

Raines was popular as the 1/5th SFG(A) surgeon. He listened to the gripes of soldiers tired of the group's deployment tempo and trained his medics as he morphed into the unit's paternalistic good-luck charm. His Special Forces A teams left Afghanistan's Tora Bora Mountains in 2001 without the loss of a soldier and returned to their busy but routine life at Ft. Campbell.

It was not until Operation Iraqi Freedom in 2003 that his good-luck-charm image began to tarnish. While securing an airfield in western Iraq during the early hours of the March 2003 invasion, one of his teams was pounded by mortar fire during a firefight, killing four 5th Group soldiers and their medic.

Although Raines knew all of these men well, his decision to leave the military after his obligated service ended came from a smaller set of horrors. The decision followed the tracks of hundreds of little blue-green balls. The little balls were the leftover components of unexploded cluster bombs, and they blew off the hands and feet of the Iraqi children who tried to play with them. As Raines looked into the anguished face of a nine-year-old left with shrapnel in his belly and chest, he felt responsible for helping to bring such a pestilence to these people. He left the Army, as a major, in 2006.

He had been an attending physician for the Jefferson Hospital emergency department for a little longer than a year and had never mentioned the things he had seen and been a part of before he arrived at the old facility. Only Karen seemed to have any knowledge of his covert past, since her husband was a retired Army colonel who still had connections.

Raines could see Karen shaking her head as she exited the triage room. He was freshly clothed in new scrubs and looked for her judgment to guide him to the next patient in need. She placed a hand on his arm and sheepishly whispered to him about the urgent needs of the next patient in triage.

"No way, Karen!" Raines quickly responded. "It's too busy. Send her down to the animal hospital on Bainbridge."

"Please, Dr. R.," she cajoled, "She won't go because she's afraid that it will bleed to death!"

Raines rolled his eyes and took a suture tray from the supply cart. Mustering more kindness than his fatigue easily offered, he stepped through the double doors into triage. Raines saw a disheveled elderly woman fearfully holding a wriggling green parakeet, dabbing at the bird's blood with an old handkerchief.

"The cat bit her foot clean off!" offered the old spinster as Raines's eyes drifted to the bloody birdcage at the woman's feet.

"Hold her feet up," Raines suggested, and the worried bird lady turned her pet's lower end to the sky, pointing one foot and one bloody stump toward the doctor. Raines deftly placed a figure-of-eight suture through and around the stump and then secured it with a surgeon's knot. The oozing of blood stopped, and the bird lady shared her near-toothless grin.

"Another one saved," Raines smiled to Christie as he retreated into the real-care world of the emergency department. As he picked up the chart for the next case, a worried mother and her feverish child, he laughed at the thought of the one-footed bird back at home in its cage, tilting crazily on the perch.

Chapter 3

INDEPENDENCE SQUARE

Philadelphia; August 2008

Raines signed over the responsibility for the remaining patients to his relief physician at seven a.m. and headed for the triage door.

"G'night, Doc," Christie called.

Raines waved and ducked through the sliding glass door into the summer morning. As he headed toward his Harley-Davidson in anticipation of a peaceful ride home, he spied Aimee's BMW in the doctors' parking lot.

"Hi, hon," Raines began.

"Hi, yourself," the young woman responded. Aimee Hargrove's long, blonde hair was usually straight, but today she wore it piled high upon her head in careful, crown-like curls. She was twenty-eight, a bit thin and less than full chested, and Raines had felt her to be glaringly self-centered on more than one occasion. Although she was dressed for work at the travel agency, the business did not open for another hour.

"What you doing out so early?" smiled Raines.

"Just wanted to make sure I didn't miss you," Aimee said, "and I'm going to pick up a grey Chanel sweater dress that I have my eye on. Its slow now at the office, so I decided to do a bit of shopping on Market Street. I really just needed to tell you that my father is flying in tonight. I think he's figured out that we live together."

"Great," Raines said, pretending to read aloud the next day's headlines. "'Boston Banker Beats Up Former Ranger to Protect Daughter's Honor!'"

"Oh, it won't be like that, Ron," soothed Aimee. "He's really just a bald teddy bear. I was hoping you would switch shifts tonight so we could take Dad to dinner."

"I'll try to work out a swap," Raines said. "But what are we going to tell your dad about our 'future plans'?"

"I think we should just tell him that we haven't decided to settle down into anything as permanent as marriage yet," replied Aimee brightly.

"That's going to go over like acne on a beauty queen," he sighed.

Ron Raines mounted the Harley and began his no longer peaceful drive to the Philadelphia waterfront. When Raines finished a shift, his focus turned to enjoying the quiet marina near his apartment on Front Street, near the Old City. Along this bend of the Delaware River waterfront, only four blocks from Carpenter's Hall, the home of the First Congressional Congress, he had found a haven where finally things seemed a little less crazy than the life he had lived for thirty-eight years.

Raines parked the Harley and rubbed his eyes as they burned with fatigue. He sat down upon his usual park bench overlooking the waterfront, and pondered the keelboats and the musical clinking of the halyards against their metal masts.

The lull of the boats bobbing on the river and the shrill calling of the seagulls as they wheeled through the early-morning mists over the marina promised an escape from a world of stress; escape from emergency rooms full of death and the memories of wars where strange people tried to kill you. As he cleared his mind of the frustrating challenges of inner-city life, sitting on the waterfront for only a few moments provided a sense of peace and provided him the calm that made sleep a possibility.

~

In a parking lot in the Historic District of Philadelphia, Aimee Hargrove deftly applied eye shadow and reviewed the results in the mirror. She gathered her Louis Vitton handbag, and her heels clicked their way to the boutique's entrance. Raines's Front Street apartment was working out nicely, she thought; it had a great view and a front-gate guard for her Beemer's safety. The Old City area had quaint little shops and restaurants sprinkled among the red brick homes that held the history of heroes and patriots. Penn's Landing and the waterfront still hosted civic events, more than three hundred years after William Penn first laid out his city squares. The marina across from the apartment displayed millions of dollars worth of pleasure boats. Best of all, she was ten minutes from the Rittenhouse Square office where she worked, and living on Front Street was free.

"I'll only be a little late," she reminded herself, as though her conscience actually cared that she had not called the travel agency about her little shopping trip en route to work.

As Aimee entered a boutique on Market Street, Marwan al-Talib sat in his cab two blocks away, on the corner of Chestnut Street. It was after morning prayers and before tourists began to circulate, his time for study and meditation, and today—his time for a new contact. On his lap sat the Holy Qur'an, and the front passenger seat held his well-worn copy of the *Hadith,* whose quotations told of the simple life of the true Prophet. At twenty-two, full of youthful energy and fiery purpose, al-Talib was prepared for God's 'True Embrace' of those in Jihad.

Al-Talib's parents remained in Syria and were proud of their son, who was a member of the Martyr's Brigade living in the United States. Talib was a slight man who felt that, although the body was a temple for service to God, the exercise of his mind was of even more value to Allah. Unlike his friends in the mosque, he remained clean-shaven to better fit into the American image of a trustworthy taxi driver.

"'Let not the unbelievers think that they can get the better of you,'" he read aloud from the Eighth Sura. "'They will never frustrate you. Against them, make ready your strength to the utmost of your power, including the steeds of war, to strike terror in the enemies of Allah.'"

He read, yet again, the Ninth Sura, which outlined the three choices left for the infidel: to convert, to pay the tax, or to meet the Sword of Islam.

"'Fight and slay the pagans where ever you find them, and seize them, and lie in wait for them in every stratagem; but if they repent and establish regular prayers and practice regular charity, then open the way for them. Allah is oft-forgiving,'" al-Talib read.

Since the infidels were so resistant to conversion, al-Talib spent more of his efforts enforcing the *Jizyah,* the monetary tax that remained one of the three survival options for the unbeliever. He charged the infidels this tax as they exited his cab, though they sometimes complained that his prices were too high. Their choices outlined in the scripture were simple.

Marwan al-Talib hated this American place with its topless bars, intoxicating drinks, and homosexuals. In America, he lived *al-Tokiya,* where he "smiled outside, but hated inside."

Al-Talib watched as a tall, professional man walked by the

cab without looking at him. Al-Talib knew that the Egyptian-born man had spent the last decade teaching computer science at Philadelphia Community College. He wore wire-rimmed glasses, an open shirt and sport coat, and walked with the confidence of someone who had important plans. The man strode down Chestnut Street toward the river without looking into the storefronts and entered a Dunkin' Dough-nuts shop at the corner. Al Talib followed the man into the coffee shop after waiting to make sure no one followed. He sat across from the professional man at the rear corner table.

"Good morning, Teacher," said al-Talib humbly in Arabic.

"Are you ready, Faithful One?" Dr. Ali Zarif asked.

"Yes ... Allah Ahkbar," responded al-Talib.

"The shipment will arrive in twenty days. Has Ahmed completed the commercial license?"

"He will sit for the examination on Thursday, Teacher."

"You will meet the other Faithful at the packing plant on the night of the transport," Zarif said.

As he sat only three blocks away from Independence Square and the crowds waiting in line to view the Plexiglas-encased Liberty Bell, Zarif was finding it difficult to wait patiently when so many targets were in plain sight. The operation would be a stunning blow against this perverted government that was run by mere men rather than by the laws of Allah.

Chapter 4

THE CONTAINER

Tehran; August 2008

The lumbering orange forklift ran roughly, but its dedicated operator had become adept at getting work from the beast long after its useful lifespan had ended. With a groan, the mechanical creature locked its padded grapple around the last of the eight storage tanks and moved it a few inches into the air. The behemoth lurched forward and began to ease its load into the right outer corner of the off-white, forty-foot shipping container. The liquid-filled tank was large—two meters high and one and a half meters wide—however, it easily joined its brother tanks within the confines of this special container. Despite the cool, dark hour of the early morning, the loading dock of the Fathu al-Shamal factory was slick with condensation on the concrete, and whiffs of sweat from the workers' exertions hung in the air.

Saleeb Farhan did not like to work before morning prayers, but the general ordered that he supervise during the pre-dawn hours of this August morning. After a final review of the shipment's position, Farhan closed the double metal doors and applied the heavy-duty padlock. From the inner pocket of his dark jacket, he removed three shipping label packets and carefully applied each in turn to the sides and doors of the container. Each packet contained a U.S. Customs Form 3299, "Duty-Free Entry of Unaccompanied Articles," and a power of attorney to allow the destination agent to interact with U.S. Customs on the shipper's behalf.

An inventory in English noted six containers of liquid fertilizer "packed by owner" at their origin in Marseilles. The company of ownership was listed as Logis Sourient, though the residents of Marseilles would not recognize the mythical French company's name or the unremarkable little house located at the company's address. The Logis Sourient conglomerate had owned the empty house for nearly two years. The company's chief executive officer, duly registered with the French government, actually lived in Syria.

Farhan slowly circled the Conex for the final time, satisfied that all had been properly prepared. Two strangers appeared on the loading dock, accompanied by one of the factory's armed guards.

"Allah Ahkbar. Good morning, Mr. Farhan," said Dr. Khalid Atoomb, who introduced himself and the grinning puppy who was his assistant. "The container is ready?" he asked.

"Yes, Doctor," smiled the dock supervisor. "We are about to load the container onto the railcar. We have arranged for guards to be posted until the shipment departs for Bandar-e-Abbas, as the general has instructed."

"What is the container's weight capacity, Mr. Farhan?" Atoomb asked.

"More than thirty thousand kilograms, Doctor," answered Farhan. "The general tells us that this special container has a doubled floor and the container's lifting hardware is quite oversized. What of such importance is contained in the tanks?"

"The tanks have only liquid fertilizer," Atoomb quickly reported.

The puzzled foreman stepped around the guard to call to the operator of the side-loading forklift that was approaching the dock. Farhan guided in the massive vehicle to ensure proper balance, and the forklift operator lifted the forty-foot container for transfer to the railcar.

∼

General Madmudiyeh did not need to hear, yet again, a briefing on the container's transit, but he allowed his operations officer to enjoy his brief moment of importance. Atoomb and the Committee of Counselors had carefully selected this time of the year in order to protect the container's temperature during its long journey. None of the men on the dock knew the destination or contents of the shipment. Only the general and his staff knew that, when it reached the coastal city of Bandar-e-Abbas and the southern port of Shahid Fajai, the shipment would be transferred onto an unmarked Islamic Republic Shipping freighter.

The Iranian port of Shahid Fajai was not the largest or most modern in the republic, but it held the most loyal followers in its management. The port manager knew only of the shipment's importance to the Committee of Counselors and thus asked no further questions.

"The places during transit of most concern," the operations officer briefed to the bored intelligence general, "are during the train transit to Bandar e-Abbas, in the Persian Gulf, and on transfer to the European Diversified ship in Marseilles. Our security is reliable at Port Shahid Fajai."

Although the shipment would leave Iran under armed military guard, containers were frequently lost in international shipping. If a container broke loose from its ship, it usually floated a few inches beneath the surface of the waves and created a collision hazard for oncoming ships.

The operations officer dutifully briefed on current piracy activities in the Gulf of Oman and the expected degree of shipping congestion in the Strait of Hormuz. The Iranian vessel would have to wait for the natural bottleneck to pass up to sixty vessels before continuing.

"There are few security risks and little potential for legal seizure in traveling through the Red Sea, the Suez Canal, and the Mediterranean, due to the container's diplomatic status, but the same legal protections do not exist on the transatlantic leg of the voyage aboard the *Sonjnafiorden*. The weather in the North Atlantic on the final leg of the voyage has been predicted to be pleasant."

The operations officer smiled as he related the most significant truth of the plan. "The American customs officials inspect only five percent of the international shipping containers entering the United States. The odds are overwhelming that our special container will reach its destination unopened."

Yes, thought Madmudiyeh, *and our sword will touch thousands in a land that refuses to listen to the Iranian Republic.*

～

Three floors beneath the Fathu al-Shamal factory, Dr. Khalid Atoomb sweated through the wait for the meeting, despite the functioning air conditioning and the near constant temperature of 25 degrees Celsius. Through two long years of gene transfers, mutation failures and gene regulation problems, the Committee of Counselors seemed a distant threat with access to more than one hundred billion rials in funding. The threat was no longer distant; it lived and breathed the purified air of the underground laboratory along with him.

Atoomb absentmindedly looked yet again through the

PowerPoint slides on his laptop computer and realized that he would have seen any mistakes on his first three reviews. He had carefully prepared the slides for the Committee of Counselors event, with enough information on the difficult science involved to justify the enormous expenditures, but not enough scientific detail to lose the audience and their patience. He counted upon the counselors hope for a change in the balance of world power.

"The counselors are waiting," snapped General Madmudiyeh, who disappeared as Atoomb gathered his computer and his courage.

It will only last for an hour, he reassured himself.

Dr. Khalid Atoomb entered the underground facility's conference room with trepidation.

"*La isha il Allah,*" he said quietly and looked down to plug the digital projector's cable into his laptop's display port.

Seated at the conference table before him were four men, only two of whom he recognized from the newspapers. Two wore graying beards and the black turban of the Mullah. Two were younger, and exhibited the still-dark beards and determined eyes of those deeply dedicated to The Cause. One of the younger men wore Western clothing.

"With your permission," Atoomb began, "I will explain Allah's work here and the tools you now have at your disposal.

"Deoxyribonucleic acid, or DNA, is the tool Allah has chosen to carry the gene information for life."

Atoomb flashed a PowerPoint diagram of the DNA helical coil. There was already a puzzled look on the face of one of the Mullahs.

Even if the project proves to be an effective weapon, thought Atoomb, *I may lose my life due to the lack of understanding!*

Chapter 5

SONJNAFIORDEN

Mid-Atlantic; August, 2008

Her fading black superstructure rose only slightly higher than the rows of shipping containers winched down to her decks. Her once-red hull now showed traces of rust at the waterline as she waddled through the dark gray mid-Atlantic swells. *Sonjnafiorden*, a four-hundred-ton Norwegian container ship, steamed southwest, with her navigation plots revealing her to be 1,400 nautical miles out of Gibraltar and a little more than a thousand nautical miles south of the Azores. She used the Atlantic north equatorial current flowing westward and only 40 percent throttle to move at a comfortable eighteen knots. The crew remained relaxed, since the weather was clear, the sea was calm, and there were more than a thousand meters of water beneath the ship. The vessel still had to traverse the longest three navigation legs of the transatlantic voyage.

Captain Lars Johannsen, a twenty-eight-year veteran captain, had completed more than half of his final year in service to European Diversified Shipping. *Sonjnafiorden* was a fine old ship and seemed to the non-sailor quite large, at more than nine hundred feet in length. She was, in fact, only a middleweight for container ships these days, compared to the post-Panamax vessels that could carry twice as much as her 5,000 twenty-foot equivalent units. On this passage, she carried more than 2,000 twenty- and forty-foot containers, carefully stacked into the holds and on deck by the cranes of expert French dockworkers.

Captain Johannsen looked up from his chart to watch the intense young man Sven at the helm.

"Well, Helmsman," said the Captain, "now you're in the air gap."

"Air gap, sir?"

"The longest, and to Churchill, the most frightening engagement of World War II was the Battle of the Atlantic," recounted the gray-haired, arthritic senior captain.

Johannsen told the young seaman that American and Canadian anti-submarine aircraft could protect merchant shipping in the western Atlantic, and aircraft from Britain and Greenland could protect at least a large part of the eastern ocean, but that in the mid-Atlantic was a gap where no protection existed from the German U-boat wolf packs. German Admiral Donitz exploited the air gap during 1941 and 1942 by sending fifty to seventy-five ships a month to the bottom of the ocean. He told of the German cryptographers who broke the radio codes used by the British admiralty, giving the U-boats ten to fifteen hours warning of the formation of a convoy leaving Liverpool.

"The German U-boat command, at Chateau Kernival in Brittany, then transmitted the coordinating instructions to the U-boat fleet using the Spruchshulüsselmaschine-M, which the British called the 'Enigma Machine,'" continued Johannsen.

"This complicated bit of hardware was able to vary a single letter into more than 20,000 possible forms and then allow decoding on the receiving end. During this 'happy time' for the U-boats, one in every twenty-five U.S and British merchant mariners lost his life at sea," said the captain.

"The deepest part of the Atlantic is over nine thousand meters deep," Johannsen said. "Here in the air gap, there is an underwater mountain range called the Mid-Atlantic Ridge. Some of these mountain peaks reach to within 5,000 meters of the surface, and in that cold, dark graveyard are the skeletons of more than 2,000 merchant vessels and warships."

"Compared to that, I guess our job is boring," the helmsman remarked.

"Thankfully, yes, Sven. But the war was hard on the Germans as well. Three-fourths of all U-boat seamen never came back home."

The captain arose, stretched his painful limbs, and remarked, "I'll be in my cabin if you need me."

The tired seaman clicked on the cabin light above the desk and settled into his well-used leather chair. He poured a large water glass full of vodka and added a single ice cube.

I am more than ready for this to be the last cruise, he thought, and he felt a strange uneasiness that he could not explain.

After thirteen days at sea, the *Sonjnafiorden* approached the Delaware Bay from the southeast. Captain Johannsen used the Immarsat telephone to call the ship's expected arrival time to the Maritel operators at both twelve and at six hours from the pilot boarding area. At three a.m. on a clear August morning, he brought the throttles to idle, and the vessel slowly stopped a mile north of lighted buoy "D."

～

"We will hold for the harbor pilot at the sea buoy," Johannsen instructed the young helmsman, "and then we'll enter the southeastern directed traffic area to Cape Henlopen."

The captain's young understudy responded with an "aye-aye" nod and double-checked the ship's GPS coordinates on the moving map display.

Lars Johannsen did not like harbor pilots, the eleventh-inning heroes who didn't seem to mind keeping a crew of twenty-six waiting for someone to captain the last eighty miles of a very long journey. The harbor pilot's salary of over 300,000 U.S. dollars per year was another source of heartburn for oceangoing captains and their shipping companies, but transportation laws required pilotage by a U.S. government–licensed pilot through the Delaware Bay and the Delaware River.

Although she was not the most modern container ship on the Atlantic, the *Sonjnafiorden* sported a new interface for the vessel tracking system and was already under the careful electronic eyes of the Philadelphia harbormaster. The *Sonjnafiorden* was fully compliant with her new international ship security certificate, and the crew was trained to spot dangerous containers and subtle attempts to foil the customs officials in their international ports of call.

The Atlantic crossing had been uneventful, with the North Atlantic weather causing only eight-to-ten-foot seas and a bit of rain. After more than 130 transatlantic trips, Johannsen had seen much worse. Many of the crewmembers loitered on deck, already anxious for their promised weekend in Philadelphia. In another twenty-four hours, they could begin to drink themselves into hope-filled contact with some American lovely.

After a three-hour wait, the helmsman spotted the black, fifty-foot boat lettered "Pilot" in white. He placed a radio call to the pilot on VHF channel sixteen.

There would be no joy in the port for Captain Johannsen, who would stay on board for the lading transfers. After customs arrived at the dock, the crew would disembark, and the U.S. longshoremen would begin their work. Two Kocks forty-ton gantry cranes would rumble over the ship, rapidly lifting a container every two minutes for the next three days and nights. The shipping company contract specified that any unloading after seventy-two hours would result in monetary penalties, thus the professional pride of the long-shoremen assured the job would be completed on time. After the containers were in the temporary storage yard awaiting transport by truck or train, they would be reloaded. Then, after a total of six days in port, the *Sonjnafiorden* would sail on its backhaul trip to the old Dutch port of Rotterdam, still the largest port in the world.

As the pilot moved the vessel into the channel between Cape May and Cape Henlopen, Captain Johannsen ran the Loadline software for a final check to avoid problems with port authorities who might be concerned about *Sonjnafiorden*'s depth in the water as she entered the forty-foot-deep channel. With a draft of thirty-two feet, his ship required a deep-water port but could go into ports that the larger Panamax vessels could not enter. The Panamax container ships could only enter the busier ports of New York and New Jersey.

Without the *Sonjnafiorden* crew's knowledge, the port facility had already screened the vessel with the high interest vessel matrix. As expected, the ship was assigned routine risk category; the higher-risk vessels this week predominantly orig-inated in the Middle East, Africa, and Columbia.

The U.S. Coast Guard and Customs met vessels from high-risk countries in the channel for an entry inspection. The Coasties heightened their scrutiny during Ramadan and the July Independence Day celebrations, but each event was now months away.

"It is a shame," chuckled Johannsen, "that the two containers of French wine could not have fallen off the ship at a place more convenient to our future."

Obligatory laughs followed on the bridge.

Chapter 6

EARLY DINNER

Philadelphia; August 2008

hristie Fellows toweled her left arm and shoulder in front of the bathroom mirror. She still thought her breasts were her best feature: large and gently affected by gravity, with a splash of freckles in the cleavage between her very pink nipples. She slipped into lacy black panties and began wriggling into her clinging, black killer dress. Walt didn't have to know that she had ordered the dress from Victoria's Secret and not purchased it on a designer's runway.

She looked sexy but chose to keep her sexual inexperience to herself. She grew up as the only daughter of a preacher in rural Mississippi, graduated from Mississippi Southern, and began her first job in the big city two years before.

Dating opportunities were rare in Lucedale, and she had worked nights as a nursing assistant during her college years.

Except for a brief high school romance with the Lucedale High trumpet player, she had never even claimed a steady boyfriend.

Walt just might be the one. At thirty-three, he was already successful in representing clients in actions against employers, car manufacturers, and even yogurt producers. Penn Law had produced his confidence, his Rolex, and his Jaguar, and Christie had never before been entertained in the upscale restaurants and bars that seemed to be his comfort zone.

They met when Walt sprained an ankle playing racquetball and took the lead in getting to know his curvaceous, scarlet-haired nurse. This was the third date, and, Christie, thought, perhaps the time for a personal decision. Her apartment doorbell rang as she applied pale lipstick.

"Hi ... you look hot!" Walt exclaimed. "Are you ready? How about Antoine's?"

Christie thought that Walt's eyes were just a bit bloodshot, but she didn't smell alcohol.

"Settled Jenkins out of court today," he said, as his eyes darted around the room as he ran his fingers through his curly dark hair. "Shoe stores should know better than to give employees flimsy little stepladders to work with. Four hundred thousand—and my commission will send us to Acapulco, if you're interested." The attorney seemed anxious to move into the events of the evening, and tapped his foot as Christie tried to follow his machine-gun rapid speech.

Christie chalked up his rapid speech to the excitement of the kill and picked up her imitation Gucci handbag.

～

Antoine's, sparsely populated since it was not yet five, provided a wonderful merlot and chateaubriand while Walt briefed Christie on the two cases he planned to settle before the end of the week.

Without a glance upward to acknowledge that the dinner

had been excellent, Walt offered the waiter his credit card. The waiter, long practiced in the care and feeding of rude patrons, bowed in respect as he took the card.

Christie thought that it might make her feel better to talk about the child they lost in the OR following the motor-vehicle accident, but Walt seemed in need of talking through his plans for the upcoming week.

"I'm sorry, sir," interjected the waiter, "but there seems to be a problem with your card."

He handed the platinum American Express to Walt and waited for the attorney to select another method of payment.

"What kind of problem?" Walt asked sharply. "I've never had any problem with this card!"

"Perhaps you would like to choose another?" suggested the waiter.

"No, I would not like to choose another! I'd like to talk to your manager!"

"Right away, sir," the waiter promised.

The manager, a balding man in his fifties whose paunch bespoke his affection for Antoine's fare, approached the table apologetically.

"I'll run the charges again, sir," he offered politely, but he returned a few minutes later with fewer apologies.

"I have called American Express, sir," the manager reported calmly, "and they are quite sure that the credit account has exceeded its maximum."

"That is … preposterous!" fumed Walt, rising to depart the table.

Christie forced some semblance of a smile and handed the manager her own Capital One card.

Chapter 7

THE BANKER

Philadelphia; August 2008

At 3:14 p.m., Elwood Hargrove's commuter plane landed at Philadelphia International, ten minutes ahead of schedule.

"With all of the airlines going bankrupt, I guess they're trying harder to please," said Ron Raines from his position behind Aimee in the arrivals lounge.

"Come on, let's hurry!" Aimee said and tugged Ron toward the deplaning passengers. Raines followed in mock cheer, less than ecstatic to ask for a day off just to shepherd the gruff old banker through the Independence Square tourist crush. They had only spoken over the phone, and even then, Raines could hear the suspicion in Hargrove's voice.

"Oh, Daddy," squealed Aimee. "It's so good to see you!"

She threw her arms around the hefty, balding man, who

looked as though he preferred a three-piece suit to his current sport shirt and slacks.

"How are things in Boston?"

"Same old grind," he shrugged. "How's my little girl?" His stern countenance relaxed for just a moment.

"We're just great!" was Aimee's overwhelmingly positive reply. "I'd like you to meet Ron Raines."

"It's a pleasure, sir," Raines said as the older man cautiously shook the offered hand.

"We have so much planned, if you aren't too tired from your flight, Daddy."

"I'm just fine, dear," he replied. "Lead on."

~

"They've beefed up security considerably since 9/11," commented Ron as the trio waited at the metal detector located in the Sansom Street security screening building in front of Independence Hall.

"Too damn much, if you ask me," Hargrove said. "They're going to discourage the tourists who want to visit Philadelphia and spend their dollars."

"Well, I can imagine the public relations value of an attack on the Liberty Bell or Independence Hall," replied Raines, who had a more intimate knowledge of the evil things that men could plan.

"What if someone bombed the First Bank of the United States?" Raines asked the older man in an attempt to relate the risks to the world that held importance to the financier.

Hargrove seemed in a hurry as the little group looked through the glass at the Liberty Bell, stopped at Franklin's grave, and then visited the National Constitution Center.

"I'll have to be going back on the eight-thirty," commented Hargrove.

Raines wondered about the right timing for the required discussion.

"We have dinner reservations if you have the time," he offered dutifully.

Aimee drove the BMW with her father in the passenger seat. They rocketed down the Delaware Expressway toward Broad Street and the cruise terminal at Pier One.

"'Nautical Breezes with a Diverse Culinary Experience'" proclaimed the banner at the gangplank of the sternwheeler the *Liberty Belle*.

"The sunset cruise will return around seven" Raines said. "You should still have plenty of time to make the flight."

The paddle wheeler's festive red, white, and blue flagging faded into twilight as the sun set low over the city's skyline. The lobster dinner was as spectacular as the fall sunset view of the historic waterfront.

Over dessert, Raines thought that the timing was right.

"Sir, about our plans for the future ..." Raines began.

"Yes, I'd like to talk about that," said the banker, whose face suddenly looked as if his bank stock had dropped. "Frankly, I had hoped for ... a merger with a more politically connected family."

The offense was not just against Raines; it struck at his father, who limped through a painful life with few creature comforts. Once he had been a scrawny child in southern Arkansas, but he had paid his dues to achieve the respect he was due.

Raines paused to retain his self-control.

"I assure you, sir," he began, "that although my family is not the largest depositor to a bank, or private counsel to the governor of Arkansas, we are respected and honest members of our country with no remorse regarding our heritage. I have also served this country at great personal risk and forged my political connections on battlefields with men who were fighting for your way of life."

Raines paused to allow the financial magnate to follow each word.

"Most importantly, your daughter and I have no current plans to marry."

Aimee sat in open-mouthed shock at witnessing a side of Raines she had never seen. This man was capable of self-defense.

~

Less than a mile away, under the looming Walt Whitman Bridge, the Packer Street Ocean Terminal tugboat nudged the *Sonjnafiorden* into docking position. The anxious crewmen were already on deck, carrying their weekend bags.

"Thank you for your assistance, Captain," smiled Johannsen to the pilot with a forced professional tone.

The U.S. Customs officers were visible on the dock, awaiting the deployment of the gangplank and the captain's permission to come aboard.

More than a thousand trips through the customs inspections of a hundred countries, thought Johannsen. *Just hurry the hell up, so I can move on to docking this barge in Rotterdam and go home for the last time.*

Chapter 8

PACKER STREET TERMINAL

Philadelphia; August 2008

After thirty-one years with U.S. Customs, Charlie Fredricks was difficult to fool. He uncovered heroin shipments in the spare tires of incoming new cars, cocaine in fuel-resistant bladders secreted in motor oil drums, and even a small Japanese man who was shipping himself to Terre Haute, Indiana. The creative Asian man supplied himself all the comforts, including a DVD player and a lounge chair, but gave a rather distinctive signature on the Integrated Container Inspection System's x-ray screen.

Fredricks was an expert in the use of ICIS. The container inspection system allowed the gamma-ray imaging of the contents of a shipping container, and Fredricks had an excellent eye for hidden goods that should not enter his country. A radiation monitoring system automatically screened for nuclear weapons material, and an optical character recognition system logged in each screened container and compared it to its customs entry documents.

The problem was the number of containers. To complete his list of over 250 containers on this August afternoon, Fredricks needed to move more than thirty units an hour. Today his trainee ran the unit, with Fredricks rather enjoying his role as experienced teacher.

An older, blue International truck pulled into the examination bay, its sparkling new container standing in stark contrast to the well-worn vehicle. The driver smoked calmly behind the wheel.

"Hey, you can't smoke out there!" Fredricks yelled through the doorway.

The driver snuffed out the cigarette and waited without complaint.

"Number A-3567458, liquid fertilizer from Marseilles, for delivery to Pine Bluff, Arkansas," Fredricks read from his screen. "Probably going to grow a few soybeans. What do you see?"

"Eight containers of liquid … no suspicious floating or submerged items in the barrels?" Fredricks's understudy offered hesitantly.

The older man studied the screen, looking for the telltale variations in the heights of the fluid in the barrels that would reveal a submerged item with the same density as the liquid fertilizer.

"Yeah, it passes," Fredericks agreed. "Next truck."

Ahmed Madawi suppressed his desire to smile, carefully dropped the International into low gear, and pulled the special container into America.

~

Ahmed Madawi slowly exited the ramp from Interstate 95 into the industrial district of South Philadelphia. The truck was more than ten years old and its blue paint fading, but it ran reliably—at least reliably enough for its single planned delivery. He drove slowly to feel out the big vehicle, even though he had been to the plant before and had become familiar with the route plotted on his map. Although no weapons were yet on board, Madawi had carefully measured the driver's-side map pocket to make sure a 9mm Uzi submachine gun would fit.

As Madawi's truck crawled past a roadside coffee shop, a Philadelphia police cruiser pulled from its parking space to follow the vehicle. Officer Hardruff thought a young Arabic male driving a rig so carefully had potential, if only for the DOT paperwork fines. After his dispatch identified the vehicle as one owned by Landers Trucking of Phoenix, Arizona, last registered in 2004, he accelerated and hit the blue lights.

Ahmed Madawi felt his heart pound when he saw the rapidly approaching cruiser, with its blue lights demanding attention. He eased the old International and its trailer to the shoulder of the industrial roadway.

"Forgive me, Officer," Madawi said politely, "have I failed to comply with the city laws?"

Without reply, the officer stepped onto the running board, tilted his sunglasses to the tip of his nose, and let his eyes roam over the truck's interior. He saw castoff McDonald's bags, cigarette packs and empty canned lemonade containers, but no visible contraband.

"License and registration, please," commanded Hardruff without a trace of hospitality despite being in the City of Brotherly Love.

Madawi reached into the glove box and retrieved the vehicle bill of sale and the 2004 Arizona registration, plus the diesel mechanic's survey of the truck, completed only two days earlier.

Lastly, and with pride, Ahmed Madawi handed over his two-week-old DOT commercial driver's license.

"What is your destination?" queried Hardruff, unable to completely hide his surprise over the production of a valid license.

"I am expected at the Arsenault Meat Packing Company," Madawi replied with growing confidence. His cell had planned the operation well.

Hardruff was familiar with the aging meat company, primarily by its smell. He avoided the area on his rounds unless he had police business in the adjacent tenements.

"Everything seems to be in order," reported Hardruff with disappointment. "Be sure that you register this vehicle with the State of Pennsylvania within thirty days."

He then stepped down from the truck, returned to his cruiser, and drove rapidly to the north.

Madawi reentered the roadway and followed the last four turns to bring him to the plant. As he piloted the tractor-trailer through the chain-link fence of the meat packing company, Ahmed Madawi thanked Allah for the preparations of his leaders.

Chapter 9

THE FAITHFUL

South Philadelphia; September 2008

The bright yellow, late-model Econoline van carried the moniker Loring Valve Company on each side, followed by an address and phone number in Thibedeaux, Louisiana. The occupants seemed in no hurry as they drove through South Philadelphia on a September evening after sunset prayers. The glove box contained the van's new bill of sale; however, the vehicle remained registered to the now defunct Loring.

Behind the wheel was Dr. Ali Zarif, a full professor at the Community College of Philadelphia, his position largely due to the publication of his papers in the field of computer encryption. Thin, quietly intelligent, taller than his Brothers and bespectacled, he was a well-respected member of the college faculty and was liked by his colleagues. Nevertheless, as did the other five men in the van, Zarif still held close the belief that the world was an evil place, laden with those who failed to see the need for religious guidance and failed to make their lives purposeful. His life would be purposeful. His deep, driving purpose was to punish the adherents of a "superpower" philosophy who believed that men could direct the decisions of other men without divine guidance.

Though Zarif was Egyptian by birth, his last visit to his homeland had been almost eight years before. Zarif's distance from the Middle East, however, did not impede his contacts in the region. Using his own computer encryption programs, he maintained contact with hundreds of members of the Brotherhood of Islamic Jihad. He alone was responsible for managing the funding that flowed from the U.S. and Middle Eastern organizations into the coffers of the Philadelphia mujahideen cell.

This evening, Zarif was dressed in dark slacks, black running shoes, and a lightweight, long-sleeved nylon pullover. By his previous orders, neither he nor the five young Faithful who shared the van wore the keffiyeh.

Stealth was the key to the operation's success; the Brothers passed as silently among the citizens as the shadows beneath a new moon. None of the mujahideen wore body armor, since they carried the armor of Allah.

"Teacher, will the Saudi royal family and the Jordanians support us in our battle?" quietly questioned Musa, a bearded Egyptian, from his seat in the van's second row.

"The royal family is composed of selfish fools, and the Jordanian government dances to the tunes of the Americans," answered Zarif. "They have not yet progressed to a fully Islamic leadership. Some feel that the governments of Egypt, Pakistan, and Turkey are Islamic, but they are false states, not Islamic republics following the true path of the prophet. I pray our actions will help to bring sister governments back to the true light and the need to govern by the laws of the Shira'a."

"Will the infidels increase their security because of the date on which we strike?" asked the one-eyed Iranian Mohammed, causing Farouk in the front passenger seat to also turn toward the teacher for his answer.

Farouk, the younger of the two Iranian brothers, wore a beard like Mohammed's and relied upon his brother to form his own opinions.

"No," replied the teacher. "Although this date is not forgotten, to the Americans this date seems a geographically and temporally distant problem. They are rats on the exercise wheel of jobs, monthly payments, and the pleasures of the flesh. They do not yet see the terrible, final nature of Allah's judgment."

"And we are the instruments of that judgment," volunteered Mohammed, whose face was seared and grotesquely scarred.

"How many workmen will we find at the sites?" asked Abdul-Wahhab from the third row of seats.

"We expect a guard and two workmen at the pumping station in Philadelphia and an empty building at the Team Two site in New York. The five-man team in Philadelphia will have no difficulties; the guard carries only a revolver," Zarif reassured him.

He went on. "The three of you in Team Two will complete your mission before the authorities are aware that you are near the city."

As the men concentrated on their assigned tasks and the grave importance of the trial at hand, they continued the remainder of the drive in silence. The van turned into the open gates of the Arsenault Meat Packing Company, where the vehicle ground to a halt on the perpetually bloodstained gravel.

Farouk and young Jafar exited and then closed and locked the gate behind them, then walked across the reddish-brown parking lot to meet the fellow Faithful.

The van proceeded to the rear of the lot, where two figures waited in the dark by the worn blue International tractor-trailer. The long-haul trailer still held the specially reinforced off-white, forty-foot container, which bore the labels indicating its Marseilles origin.

"*A'-Salam Aley'kum*; may peace be with you" offered Zarif as the group exited the van.

"*Wa-Aley'kum as-Salam*; and peace to you, also," responded Marwan al-Talib and Ahmed Madawi from the shadows near the truck.

Dr. Zarif produced the keys to the heavy brass padlock on the loading dock's double doors. The Faithful followed the path of thousands of doomed cattle across the loading dock and through the threshold into the dimly lit, cavernous old factory.

Madawi expertly backed the International and its special cargo to the loading dock, releasing a rain of rust from the plant's roof as the trailer nudged into position.

In the center of the plant, between the pools of stagnant water on the worn, irregular concrete, waited a modified three-quarter-ton pickup truck. The truck, brought at a city surplus sale in Des Moines, Iowa, retained its rusty green paint and the city emblem that was now too faded to read. Although both of the old truck's doors creaked, and the bench seat was cracked, hemorrhaging its foam padding, the vehicle was not neglected. During the year of its residence at the factory, the engine had been tuned, and the truck had received a new, quieter muffler and a dark green canvas bed enclosure to shield the cargo area from the weather and prying eyes. Where once rusty shovels had lain just behind the cab, now vital equipment rested.

An expensive, industrial-grade water pump had been bolted into the truck bed, and its seven-horsepower electric motor was coupled to an 800-watt AC inverter by cables running through the truck cab. The truck also now held an auxiliary battery in the cab, a battery large enough to supply 110-volt power to its pump for more than eight hours.

As Madawi and al-Talib broke the seals and opened the doors of the container, Abdul-Wahhab started a nearly new forklift and approached the rear of the container. Madawi guided him into position, and Abdul-Wahhab closed the grapple-arms of the powerful beast around the rearmost tank in the shipping container.

"Put the outer six here," motioned Zarif, even though just above the selected spot the stars were visible through the dilapidated metal roof.

Abdul-Wahhab set down the tank with a jolt and returned for another.

After the four outer tanks had been removed, the forklift entered the shipping container with significantly greater care. Abdul-Wahhab carefully lifted one of the remaining two tanks, and the beast slowly backed out, pivoted, and placed it into the bed of the aging green truck.

Al-Talib put on a pair of bright orange dishwashing gloves and began to connect the fitting on the base of the special tank resting in the pickup truck to the six-inch flexible stainless-steel hose that led to the inlet side of the new pump. He closed the tank's valve and double-checked the pump's outlet connections to the four-inch rubberized hose that coiled, massive and snakelike, over most of the remaining bed space. Satisfied that the tank was properly attached to its delivery system, he rose to face Zarif.

Zarif gave a single nod, then entered the shipping container and knelt beside its lone remaining fertilizer tank. He removed a panel from the metal floor, and reached beneath the container's floor level, where his hand found the goods hidden in a four-inch deep, lead-lined compartment. The Faithful stood anxiously as he unwrapped each of the six new AK-74M rifles and handed them in turn to his understudies. He then removed two Soviet-issue Ruchnoy RPG-7 anti-tank missiles, and finally, four Makarov PMM 9mm pistols. Zarif handed up thirty-round banana clips for the AK weapons, six AK silencers, and four Soviet RGD-5 hand grenades. The hidden compartment was empty after he removed the four boxes of 9mm pistol ammunition and eight boxes of 5.45 rounds for the rifles. Zarif smiled, as his Faithful young men excitedly examined the weapons and retreated from the container.

Abdul-Wahhab's forklift then lined up on a wooden pallet that held a second industrial-grade pump and scooped it from the factory floor. He carefully maneuvered the loaded pallet into the shipping container and placed the device near the remaining tank. Ahmed Madawi entered the container with his gloves and tools and connected the tank to the inlet side of the heavy new pump. Mohammed and Musa manhandled the fifty-foot, heavy-duty outlet hose into the container, where Madawi took charge of its installation as well.

"Before Team Two departs, let us have tea and pray," Zarif said quietly.

Zarif sat before a battered coffee table and lit the propane flame on a small, portable stove. After warming the tea that they would share, he poured the fluid into small glasses and fortified each glass with several spoonfuls of sugar. As Zarif shared the tea, the eight dedicated men waited for midnight and for the opportunity to perform their duties during the early morning hours of September 11th.

Chapter 10

YONKERS

Interstate 95 North; 10 September 2008

Young Jafar lit an unfiltered Camel cigarette and looked to Marwan al-Talib, who piloted the tired green municipal pickup along the darkened interstate.

"You promised that you would give us the Team Two plan after we left Philadelphia," he said.

"As I shall," announced al-Talib, relishing his position of trust. *Our target is so much simpler than Philadelphia,* he thought as the old green truck sped north along Interstate 95.

Abdul-Wahhab carefully shifted his feet to avoid the large storage battery resting on the floorboard.

"The city does not depend on water treatment, since the Catskill and Delaware watershed areas naturally filter the water for them," al-Talib began. "The city leaders are still fighting the national government to avoid the expense of a water treatment plant. Only chlorine and soda ash are added to the water, in three different locations, before the people use it.

"We drive north of the city, and approach the Hillview reservoir through the Yonkers Raceway," al-Talib continued. "Over the past year, the reservoir has been covered for additional security, but all of the Department of Environmental Protection's recent care and attention has been upon the new water tunnel, Number Three, under construction for the city. While they tunnel their expensive new project 800 feet deep in the New York bedrock, no one watches the older Tunnel Number One, which still carries more than a third of the water to the city."

"So how do we gain access to the tunnel?" probed Jafar.

"Six shafts reach down from the surface to the old 1917 tunnel," continued al-Talib, "and three of them are in unguarded gatehouses where the chlorine is stored."

Al-Talib looked closely at young Jafar to gauge his readiness to carry out the plan as he had been instructed.

"We attack Shaft 22, in a city park area just south of the reservoir, and need to defeat only a single lock. We will use the locksmith tool to enter the gatehouse, and then we will pass in about twenty feet of the four-inch hose."

Al-Talib waited but heard no discussion from his two assistants.

"If this truck holds up, we will be in the gatehouse by one a.m., and by three o'clock, the blessing will be on its way to the buildings of Manhattan."

~

At one a.m., the alarm on Dr. Ali Zarif's watch punctuated the silence of the packing plant with three short beeps.

"It is time for us to take our place in the world history of our faith," the teacher said simply.

The four Faithful sat cross-legged on grimy rugs surrounding the small table that held their flame. In each man's hand was an AK-74M, now with a thirty-round clip in place and fitted with the silencer that would mute the weapon's fire to the sound of a dull saw chewing through old wood.

The Faithful took their appointed places in the Loring Valve van that waited at the loading dock. Zarif avoided placing the padlock on the plant's rear double doors; he had no plan to return and he was confident that an open door indicated there was nothing worth seeing in the old slaughterhouse.

Zarif looked at each face in the van, and when no man's countenance registered fear or indecision, he pulled the lever into drive and slowly exited the rusty brown driveway.

Chapter 11

PUMPING STATION A

Philadelphia; 11 September 2008

ong before Europeans interfered in their peacefulness, the
Nantichoke and Minqua groups of the Delaware Indians
lived along a river that slowly snaked from its watershed in
present-day New York through rolling hills, green glens, and
granite cliffs over four hundred miles to the sea. In 1631 Dutch
proprietors formed the Dutch West India Company and
settled into the region beyond the Delaware Capes.

The English seized the Dutch holdings along the river,
and claim to the area transferred from the English Duke of
York to William Penn in 1682. Penn used the Delaware River
to demarcate the Quaker colony of Pennsylvania from New
Jersey and New York.

The Delaware carried striped bass, channel catfish and
mussel hatchlings, in addition to coalmine discharges, pesti-

cides, and chlorinated biphenyls from sewage treatment plants. Yet the river was the source of drinking water for more than seventeen million people. To comply with the Safe Drinking Water Act, the Delaware River politicians established an elaborate process for purifying their water.

The raw water flowed in from the river and underwent purification at one of three water treatment plants. Over half of the city's supply was purified at the Baxter Water Treatment Plant facility. At the Baxter Plant, over 200 million gallons of raw water daily sat in settling ponds before being filtered by a sand filtering system. The water was treated with ferric sulfate and calcium oxide; checked for bacteria, heavy metals, phosgene, radiation, and the byproducts of the industrial areas to the north. The water underwent chlorination and confirmation of its clarity. The purified water was as clean as it could be made by man.

The purified Philadelphia water traveled by the city's ancient system of cast-iron mains to a service area of more than 130 square miles. A series of pumping stations maintained water pressure sufficient to serve the more than 1.5 million customers in the area.

The night shift had just begun at the Baxter Water Treatment Plant. The engineers were relaxed, since the systems for the production of water had performed flawlessly for thousands of routine shifts.

Two miles away, Pumping Station A received its clean water from the purification plant and pushed the vital fluid along predetermined routes to meet the needs of 60 percent of the city's populace. The pumping station's crew of three watched the pressure gauges, took the required samples of clean water, and continued the preventative maintenance of the pumps and lines needed to ensure the system's continued functionality for many years.

Jack Day, the operator on duty, had been a Philadelphia Water employee for twenty-two years. He was plump and gray-haired, and an avid gardener who anxiously awaited his retirement in two years.

Roger Herman, a twenty-five-year-old apprentice operator and jazz musician, dutifully followed him through the early morning hours and learned his new trade, despite the requirement that all tasks were to be done Jack's way.

"When's the wedding, Roger?" Day asked.

"She planned it for April, but I'm just going with the flow," smiled the rail-thin young man with the ponytail and earring.

"Well, if you're letting her make all the decisions, you've already learned the most important lesson of marriage," Day commented. "You know what Sam Kinison said? 'I don't worry about wars … I've been married!'"

"How long you been married, Jack?" asked Herman.

"My whole life," grinned the older man. "Marriage is a wonderful institution, you know."

"Yeah, yeah, but who wants to live in an institution, right?"

At two a.m., Jack recorded the outgoing flow levels in the six main lines and turned to his young shadow.

"How about pizza and a movie?" he offered.

"Beats working."

The operator placed the pizza in the control room microwave and then slipped *Independence Day* into the control room's DVD player.

~

At the Pumping Station A guard shack, Paul Armentrout leafed through his well-worn *Field and Stream*. At sixty, but still muscular and capable of handling security problems, Armentrout had carried a Smith & Wesson .38 for nearly three decades. Tonight, his mind was on his early-morning visit with his granddaughter, who was quite excited about their planned trip to the Valley Forge Park.

She's just a sponge at this age, he thought. *I got to make sure the right things get poured in.*

Armentrout had been a twenty-four-year-old infantryman during Vietnam, and he still flew the flag on his front porch beam.

~

Prentiss Smith hated night shift at the pumping station, but the benefits of Philadelphia city employment outweighed the pain.

"No one man should be changing these valves alone," he groused as he lifted the eighty-pound iron gate valve back into alignment with its feeder line. After he completed the tightening of the eight flange bolts and lock nuts, he was going to take a smoke break. The muscles rippled beneath the smooth black skin of Smith's right arm as he read the numbers on the torque wrench's tension gauge. The arm had almost taken him to better places. He had been one hell of a pitcher fifteen years before, and Penn State had offered him a scholarship. He had decided to leave college to support his new family when his girlfriend became pregnant. Now his daughter was a sophomore at Philadelphia Community College.

Just after two a.m. on the Day of Jihad, a deadly caravan moved slowly through the Arsenault company gates and proceeded with careful attention to the traffic laws of Philadelphia's Torresdale area. Dr. Ali Zarif was at the wheel of the Loring Valve van, as his brother Mohammed, Farouk, and Egyptian Musa rode quietly in the rear seats. Following at a careful distance was the ancient blue International, driven with grim determination by Ahmed Madawi.

As instructed, the tractor-trailer stopped on the road's shoulder half a block from the Philadelphia Water Department's Pumping Station A. The yellow Loring Valve van entered the fenced gate and stopped at the guard shack.

Although it was a strange hour for a service call, Paul Armentrout knew that Prentiss Smith sweated alone with a set of valve replacements in the station. He walked to the van driver's window to see a smiling professorial type extending a sheaf of property papers.

"Good morning, Paul," said Ali Zarif, with the papers extended in his left hand.

Armentrout looked closely at the face without recognition but assumed that the service call was probably at the correct location. As Armentrout accepted the paperwork and looked down, Zarif's right hand rapidly moved forward, accurately placing the half-million-volt stun baton against the guard's chest. Zarif fired.

Armentrout managed only a grunt of pain and a look of wide-eyed shock before he slumped in total muscle failure. Dr. Ali Zarif prevented his fall into the gravel, and Farouk rapidly exited of the van's sliding side door.

Wordlessly, Farouk heaved the inert grandfather into the rear of the van, which then slid unimpeded into the pumping station parking lot. Farouk bound Paul Armentrout with duct tape around the hands, feet, and mouth, and left him to fear the results of his failure to protect the station in his charge.

The yellow van ground to a halt as the blue International began to pull its load into the parking lot. The tractor-trailer halted squarely in front of the large bay doors of the facility, blocking the line of vision into the building from the nearby street.

Zarif and the three Faithful from the van moved rapidly into the brilliantly lit interior of the pumping station's open central bay. As Zarif moved around the building's inner perimeter and provided cover, Mohammed kicked open the control room door and rushed inside, followed by Farouk and Musa.

Day and Herman jumped from chairs in open-mouthed amazement, pizza still in hand, as the three terrorists stood near the control panel and then fired on the operators, television and control panel. The 5.45-millimeter rounds chewed into fragile human chest, abdomen, and neck and then puffed out inside, forming ragged-edged projectiles of death. The three short bursts from the silenced AK's had sealed the fate of the room's unbelievers in less than four seconds.

From his pipeline work area, Prentiss Smith heard no vehicles or gunfire but saw much more movement than was to be expected near the control room. Still clutching his twelve-inch torque wrench, he moved to the control room door to investigate. Just as Smith's hand touched the knob, the door burst open, revealing the three men exiting and the carnage inside the room.

"What the hell?" spat Smith as the armed men froze momentarily in surprise. In that instant, forty-two years of pent-up frustration rode the arc of Smith's wrench, and his muscular arm swung it onto the top of the head of the first man through the door.

Musa dropped without consciousness of his fatal injury. He only remembered that he was doing something of great importance, as his failing mind recalled his mother and the goats standing in the baked mud yard of his home in western Iraq. His vision of home then faded into darkness.

The burst from Zarif's silenced AK-74 was only as loud as the annoying buzz of a swarm of bees, but the twenty rounds hit Prentiss Smith in the back and head with devastating results. A spray of blood and fragments of bone peppered Mohammed and Farouk, who still stood shocked in the control room door. Fewer than two minutes after the van's arrival, Allah controlled Pumping Station A.

Paul Armentrout struggled as Mohammed hauled him roughly from the van, then summarily dragged him into the light of the station's interior. He saw the professorial-looking man standing beneath the station's large bay door, motioning for someone to back a vehicle into the spacious entrance. It was the last thing that he saw before two rounds from a Makarov 9mm entered the back of his skull.

Madawi jumped down from the truck and threw open the off-white container doors. He pulled forty feet of the rubberized hose from the container's interior and dragged it toward the right side of the station interior. Team One's intimate knowledge of the station's blueprints made finding the first of the inspection valves an easy task. Through the heavy-duty sight glass of the inspection valve, he saw the purified, clear water as it flowed toward the feeder mains that exited the pumping station.

Madawi twisted the iron wheel that closed the purified water line that led into the inspection valve.

"This is surely God's work," said Madawi as he removed the stainless-steel bolts that secured the inspection plate onto the top of the valve. With gloved hands, he attached the flange of the rubberized connector hose to the top of the inspection valve and replaced the bolts, securing the container's deadly cargo to the station's elaborate system of pipes.

"It is prepared," announced Madawi. Farouk nodded and climbed onto the bumper of the blue International and inside the container. Zarif nodded his authorization, and Farouk opened the tank's valve and threw the single switch that controlled the container's new pump. The quiet electric motor began to power the container's pump at almost seven hundred liters per hour, with each throb transmitting the wrath of Allah to unsuspecting infidels.

Zarif helped Mohammed load the freshly departed body of their comrade Musa into the shipping container.

"Our brother died in Jihad," Zarif reminded Mohammed. "He is already in paradise. He will be buried without washing so that Allah will see the blood of his Faithfulness."

Zarif glanced at his watch and calculated the time required for completion of emptying the container into the feeder lines. The Faithful would be ready to depart the facility around five a.m., two full hours before the next shift would arrive. After pumping the container dry, the blessing would then be on the way to the faucets of 60 percent of Philadelphia's citizens.

Chapter 12

HILLVIEW RESERVOIR

Yonkers, New York; 11 September 2008

At 1:20 a.m., Marwan al-Talib and his Team Two assistants left Interstate 95, crossed the Hudson River at Fort Lee, and continued northward on the Major Deeson Expressway. They turned the old green truck into the frontage road by the Yonkers Raceway toward the south end of the ninety-acre manmade lake.

Al-Talib turned the truck into a small park with concrete walkways that paralleled the darkened reservoir. He parked the vehicle in front of an old brick gatehouse with stone pelicans and intricate scrollwork carved into the supports above the door. The doubled doors of the gatehouse were of glass and aluminum, secured by a heavy, stainless steel chain and padlock. Al-Talib thought it ridiculous to have such sturdy hardware providing one's peace of mind when the door itself was only glass. He did not bother with the locksmith tool and merely kicked out the right lower panel of glass.

"Let's move it in," he encouraged, and Jafar and Abdul-Wahhab began pulling the four-inch rubberized tool of destruction through the open panel into Shaft 22.

Three miles away, the Yonkers Police Department alarm alerted a sleepy second-year officer assigned to the grave-yard shift. A new camera system, purchased with Homeland Security grant funds only three months earlier, rested in the elaborate stonework and now broadcast the presence of three individuals at the old Tunnel One access site.

"That looks like more than teenage pranksters," said the shift supervisor. "Call out the team."

The dark blue SWAT van swerved through the frontage road of the racetrack, trailed by two Yonkers City Police units without lights and sirens. The three vehicles entered the south Hillview Reservoir Park, and slid to a halt just out of the view from the inside of Shaft 22's glass doors. Six SWAT members with MP-5 submachine guns rushed the doorway as the Yonkers PD units assumed watch positions.

Inside, al-Talib completed the connection of the pump's outlet hose to the sight glass on the Shaft 22 plumbing and nodded to Jafar to start the pump. Young Jafar ducked through the aluminum frame of the doorway where the glass had been kicked free and raised his face directly into the aim of four submachine gun muzzles. His AK-74 still leaned against the wall back inside of the shaft, and furthermore, he was not sure that he would have fired it at them. Jafar simply raised his empty hands.

Without a word from the SWAT sergeant, team members ratcheted handcuffs tightly onto Jafar's wrists, pulled him away from the gatehouse entrance, and shoved him, face-down, into the back of a Yonkers police cruiser

"You are surrounded!" the SWAT sergeant barked through the broken glass. "Raise your hands and exit the building!"

Abdul-Wahhab's eyes flew open wide as he turned to his leader in panic. Marwan al-Talib crawled across the concrete to the center of the gatehouse with his assault rife held out before him. He rolled onto his left side, tugged his single Russian grenade from a windbreaker pocket, and held the circular pin between his teeth. Al-Talib pulled the grenade away from its pin and tossed the deadly metal egg though the broken doorframe and onto the sidewalk outside.

"Grenade!" warned a voice outside, two long seconds before the concussion blew down the remainder of the aluminum doorframe and hurled shrapnel into the waiting police cruisers and the legs of the two SWAT team members who had not yet taken cover. The two stricken officers, protected by Kevlar vests and helmets, dropped to the sidewalk, moaning in pain … yet quite alive.

Al-Talib followed the grenade's blast through the destroyed door, walking slowly while firing short, silenced bursts from the AK-74 held at his waist level. His shots shattered the windshield of one of the Yonkers cruisers and peppered the two injured officers lying prone on the sidewalk with razor-sharp shards of glass.

Simultaneously, four of the SWAT members fired their submachine guns from positions of cover, striking al-Talib in the neck and chest. The terrorist leader did not even look surprised as he fell lifeless onto the sidewalk.

Faced with the reality of the firepower waiting outside, Abdul-Wahhab abandoned his weapon, raised his hands, and stepped into the glare of the police car headlights trained on the remnants of the doorway.

"I am not armed!" he cried out, stepping forward while turning his head away from the machine gun bursts he expected to feel.

"On the sidewalk!" commanded the SWAT sergeant. "Face down … arms and legs spread!"

Abdul-Wahhab complied, and lay beside al-Talib's motionless body. The officers slammed handcuffs into place on Abdul-Wahhab's writs, as two SWAT team members began to search the gatehouse for any remaining hostiles.

The SWAT sergeant lifted the green canvas cover over the old truck's bed. He looked puzzled when he saw the metal tank and the length of monster-sized rubber hose that filled the bed of the truck.

"Better call out the chief," he said. "I got no idea who to call to start identifying all this stuff."

Chapter 13

THE AFFECTED

Philadelphia; 11 September 2008

"See you tonight, Dr. R.," Karen called as Ron Raines departed triage for the parking lot.

"Thanks for your help. See you tonight," smiled Raines as he slipped the cycle jacket onto his shoulders. The grave-yard shift had been as stressful as usual, with a twelve-year-old presenting DOA after being hit by a car and an AIDS patient dying from the toxoplasmosis that infected his brain. Perhaps no one would die when he returned tonight.

Ron entered the apartment to an inviting smile from Aimee, who was getting ready for work.

"Have time for a shower?" she winked.

"Appealing ... but I'm just too bushed," Ron responded, kissing her forehead and heading for the bedroom. He settled onto the bed and picked up the medical journal that would act as his morning soporific. He had been asleep only a few minutes when he awakened to Aimee's frightened call for help.

Ron groggily dashed into the bathroom, where he found Aimee naked and seated on the cold tile floor.

"What happened?" Ron began, but stopped short when he saw that her shoulders slumped weakly forward and she was unable to speak. Her small breasts heaved with her rapid, shallow breaths and he saw a look of pure terror carved onto her face.

Her hands flickered, and her right eye was nearly closed. *This is bad,* he thought, *but why would she stroke at twenty-eight? She's not a cocaine user and not even a smoker.*

Ron gently lay Aimee back, placed a dry towel beneath her head, and covered her with her fur-lined robe.

"Does your head hurt?" he asked, but she only stared forward, with twitches of motion in both hands, but unable to speak.

"I'm calling for help," Ron reassured her and ran for the bedroom phone.

Ron reached the EMS dispatcher after what seemed to be several minutes.

"I need an ambulance stat … 2314 North Front Street, Apartment 4300." He spoke with relatively well-controlled urgency.

"We'll do the best we can," responded dispatch. "We've had an unbelievable number of calls and have units responding from Darby and even from Camden, across the river."

Although the conversation puzzled Raines, Aimee needed his attention.

Raines returned to Aimee's side and wondered if he should call her parents. *I really don't know them very well,* he rationalized. He decided to call from the emergency department after her CT scan.

As Ron comforted her, Aimee's eyes revealed her terror,

and tears welled up in the corners of her unmoving eyes.

Oh, hell, Ron's mind blared, *this is really, really, a bad thing.*

He caressed her cheek and told her he would take care of her. The doctor in Raines felt for a pulse, and he found her carotid artery bounding rapidly in her paralyzed desperation. He wondered if she had enough swelling inside her skull to cause breathing problems, and wished he kept emergency equipment in a bag at home.

Just support her and wait, Raines reasoned, wishing for the ambulance and the comfort of an emergency department and CT scanner.

He heard the gurney near the door before the doorbell rang.

"It's open," he yelled.

Two paramedics rushed into the room, pushing a gurney loaded with a medical box and defibrillator.

"I'm an ER doc," Raines explained. "She's twenty-eight, no health problems or allergies, presenting a sudden paralysis and inability to speak."

The senior medic opened the medical toolkit, slapped on a blood pressure cuff, and checked Aimee's pupils and respiration.

The senior paramedic's name was Fields, and Raines found himself oddly fixated on the medic's metallic nametag, forced to learn the name of a man he would rather meet in more pleasant circumstances. Fields knelt by Aimee's head and softly placed a hand on her cheek.

"Ma'am," he comforted, "we're going to get you over onto a transport gurney and to the hospital. Don't worry; we'll take care of you."

Field's assistant had connected an oxygen mask to a portable tank and placed the mask over Aimee's pale lips and the small beads of sweat forming upon her face. After connecting a tiny pulse oximeter to Aimee's index finger, the junior medic rolled the lowered gurney beside her paralyzed body. The medics lifted her together and secured her with straps across her chest, abdomen, and legs.

"We're ready, Doc," Fields said. "To University?"

"No, to Jefferson," responded Raines as he numbly followed the EMS team to the apartment door.

⌒

Within ten minutes, the Medstar ambulance neared the Jefferson Hospital ER. From his perch in the rear of the vehicle, Raines could see the hospital through the windshield. The scene that appeared to be an unfolding caldron of chaos. Beneath the ambulance bay were six ambulances, haphazardly parked and still running. The adjacent ambulance parking area was packed with more than a dozen units from metropolitan Philadelphia, plus units from nearby cities.

As Raines watched in amazement, two privately owned vehicles screamed into the parking lot, flashing desperate emergency lights and attempting to get as close to the ER doors as possible. The drivers of both cars jumped from their vehicles to run into the triage area. A LifeFlight helicopter was preparing to land in the grass, since its pad was now crowded with the cars, trucks, and vans that spilled over from the hospital's parking lot. Traffic approaching the hospital had slowed to a crawl and then stopped as the crush of frightened people descended upon the facility.

"Something is very, very wrong," mumbled Raines with growing concern.

The medics looked at each other, and unable to reach the hospital, they shrugged and moved into Plan B. They pulled the ambulance onto the sidewalk alongside Chestnut Street and unloaded Aimee's gurney. The medics jogged as they pushed the gurney toward the hospital. Raines ran without even a glance at the sidewalk; intent instead upon watching the pounding pulse in Aimee's neck and the rhythmic rush of air from the medic's Ambu bag into her lungs. Panting, they pushed through the crowd near the doors and entered triage.

Although Raines had experienced the worst in inner-city gunshot wounds and wrecks, cared for friends dying on foreign battlefields, and even waded in to care for destroyed humans following the Afghan army's misadventure onto a land mine, Dr. Ron Raines had never seen a scene such as that before him.

Dozens of people packed the triage area, some lying on gurneys and even more lying on the floor. More than a dozen ventilators pumped oxygen into the lungs of patients with endotracheal tubes, and staff members with Ambu bags venti-lated dozens more. Individuals too weak to stand packed the chairs and floors of the waiting area. Raines could see the hallway that led to the OR, lined with rows of the cold and dead, only a small percentage of whom were covered with sheets.

"Thank God you came to help," gushed Dr. Matt Kindred as he ran by with a dozen endotracheal tubes stuffed in the rear pocket of his scrubs. "I don't know what the hell this is—some sort of toxic exposure, I guess ... but we've been in absolute hell for the last twenty minutes, and they're still pouring in."

Dr. Kindred didn't recognize that the figure on the gurney entering the emergency department was Raines's live-in lover.

Raines turned and, in surprise, found the day-shift triage nurse and Jefferson Hospital's nursing supervisor looking at him as though they expected a solution.

Although torn between his responsibilities to Aimee and his ability to assist in an emergency, Raines mentally moved rapidly into medical survival mode.

"I'll set up a forward triage in the parking lot," he offered, "and I'll need all the ET tubes and hands to bag people that you can find. And for God's sake, call EMS dispatch and try to find out what's going on!"

Without taking time to change into scrubs, Raines grabbed a crash cart and rolled it through the ambulance bay doors and onto the parking pad beyond. Nurse Christie Fellows and respiratory therapist Aphry Olaf followed him. He found a thirty-by-sixty-foot rectangular spot that was free of vehicles and locked the wheels of the crash cart into position.

"Open the mass casualty supply kit and have the guards put the triage flag up to direct the patients here," he suggested to Christie.

"Hey!" Raines yelled to the overwhelmed guard who stood watching the throng push into the ER. "Send them here... and send the ones with breathing trouble first." The guard nodded and began to direct the push of frightened people into a pair of lines leading into the new forward triage area.

Three Philadelphia Fire paramedics, who had the judgment to see that the crowd would quickly swamp the senior medical officer on the scene, quickly joined Raines. The emphasis of the emergently formed team was stabilizing each patient's airway and keeping alive those too weak to breathe. There were no gurneys outside, and the worst of the affected dropped to the concrete where they stood.

As the stream of distressed humanity slowly diverted toward his tiny island of care, Raines filled both his rear pockets with endotracheal tubes from the crash cart. In a desperate flurry of activity, the physician and his paramedic colleagues moved close to the faces of dozens of victims, feeling for each person's breath as they lay upon the unforgiving concrete. Time after time, they found pulses but inadequate breathing and quickly passed a life-saving endotracheal tube through the vocal cords into the patient's lungs. The respiratory therapist followed the physician and medics and showed each frightened family member how to attach an Ambu bag to help their loved one breathe.

"I don't know how to do that!" Olaf heard repeatedly.

"Then they will die," was her simple response.

After the Ambu bags ran out, Olaf showed family members how to breathe mouth to endotracheal tube to keep their loved ones alive until more equipment arrived.

The ashen gray faces, the absence of pulses, and the glazed, dead eyes of the dozens of those far beyond assistance caused Raines to move even more quickly to successive patients. Too many times, Raines shook his head, and the growing numbers of Philadelphia police officers and firemen on the scene would drag the bodies into an adjacent, rapidly filling hallway, as shocked family members tried to take in the horrible scene they could not comprehend.

The single hospital chaplain on duty valiantly tried to comfort, although the numbers of the grieving would have easily busied an entire seminary of pastors. Within an hour, representatives from more than twelve area churches arrived to assist at this hospital alone.

Raines had just passed a breathing tube into an expensively attired, white-haired matron with a large diamond on her left hand. Her elderly husband, in a thin tie loosened at the collar, knelt with wide eyes at the sight of his wife of fifty-three years so near death. His hands shook as Raines patiently took them and placed them on the Ambu bag that meant her survival. Their small white poodle licked the elderly woman's right hand and whined.

"Squeeze the bag every three seconds" was the sum total of instruction Raines gave the shaken man. The man nodded with determination; his wife's welfare was in his hands even more than it had been each day for the last half-century.

Raines rapidly rose from the elderly woman and nearly knocked over the television cameraman hovering inches above him.

"Kelly Crockett, Channel Six Action News!" blared the voice of a young woman in front of the camera. "Would you comment on what is happening here today?" she asked Raines.

Although Raines was angered by the reporter's inconceivably selfish request, he just said "Later," and returned to his patient's needs.

Raines turned rapidly to the next needy patient. Truth be told, he knew what was happening, and knew because he had seen it before. The paralysis, the difficulty breathing, and the curious eye weakness were symptoms he had seen in a Bedouin traveler in Afghanistan—a Bedouin traveler with a wound infected with *Clostridium botulinum,* the germ that caused Botulism!

Chapter 14

ORDEAL

Philadelphia; 11 September 2008

I*'m gonna get out of this,* thought Robert "Fuzzy" Walker as he shivered, although the East Philadelphia air was only a bit cool on this fall morning. The three tattered men stood around the orange and blue flames of the scrap wood that slowly burned in a rusted fifty-five-gallon drum. Fuzzy took a long drink of the table wine and coughed until his eyes were red and watering. He passed the bottle to Wild Will and watched him wipe off the top twice before taking his drink.

"Pretty mean cough ya got there, Fuzzy." commented Will.

"Not sure I can make it on the street this winter," Fuzzy said quietly. "Blood's been thin since Vietnam."

He pulled the tattered blue peacoat tightly around his thin chest and decided to put off going into the Old City until later in the day. He coughed more if he stayed out in the cool morning air, and there would be more tourists in the afternoon, anyway.

"I'm gonna get under the bridge, boys," nodded Fuzzy to his comrades. He shuffled toward the Franklin Bridge, with the loose sole of his right shoe making the walk difficult.

I'm gonna get it together, he promised himself. *Stop the drinking ... get some clothes, shave ... and then make some real money doing chopper work.*

He had been the best of the Huey mechanics in Da Nang, always able to make the workhorse helicopter fly with purloined parts and persistence. During Vietnam, he had been an army staff sergeant with eight years in service, and he had even entertained the thought of doing twenty.

Things changed during the war. The daily mortar attacks, the kids who dropped satchel charges on their liberators, the frustration over the lack of mechanics, and the rarity of helicopter parts—plus the isolation of the nights—combined and induced a pattern of evening drinking that he felt relieved his stress. In fact, his mornings became fuzzy, and his odor let his few friends in on the truth. By four o'clock he would get the shakes, and he had a couple to bridge the gap until his lonely night began.

When he returned from Vietnam, he worked a series of auto mechanic jobs and tried to keep his wife happy. Laura thought their daughter was perfect, an eight-year-old piano prodigy. Fuzzy Walker knew that she was a brat and almost completely devoid of musical talent.

"The piano teacher complained that we're three months behind!" Laura repeatedly pointed out.

"Eight to five and the carpool life is somebody else's dream," Fuzzy told the bourbon. After all, he had lived through hell and survived. In 1989, he left his Minnesota family life in search of his peace of mind. He sold refrigerators, worked an oilrig, and lived the glamorous life of a security guard.

"Some smartass always wants to help with my problem," he told the bourbon. "What the hell do they know about where I've been and what I've done?" Over fifteen years, his life slowly evolved into only East Philly and the train yards in the industrial areas along the river off Columbus Boulevard.

I'll get rehydrated, get some sleep, and wake up stronger, he thought through his fatigue and chills. He stopped at the Community Fountain, really just a faucet and hose by track eight. The old boxcars on the track had waited patiently for nearly a decade but had never been moved. Their paint was now peeling, their lettering was no longer legible, and their heavy steel wheels were caked with rust. It was unlikely that anyone in a position of power would notice or harass the tenement's residents near track eight.

The wine always gave Fuzzy a horrible morning thirst, and he drank his fill of the cool but slightly cloudy water from the rusty pipe near an ancient caboose. Within three minutes, he knew something was wrong. His arms and legs felt as heavy as lead, his vision blurred, and he found himself on his knees, unable to rise. He heard Will in the far distance ask if he was all right, but his reply would not leave his mouth. He found himself unable to remain on his knees, and he slumped onto his right side in a fetal position. He noted with great mental clarity that he could not breathe and wondered why he could do nothing about it. Four minutes after Fuzzy Walker's simple act of relieving his thirst, his world darkened and then ended.

~

Two hours into his furious attempt to save the victims of the ordeal, Dr. Ron Raines found himself surrounded by a sea of patients that threatened his capacity to move from his current footsteps. Over a hundred of the affected were receiving breathing support with endotracheal tubes, and almost all remained in the parking lot, lying on jackets, on the grass, or on the unforgiving concrete. Frightened family members dutifully squeezed the Ambu ventilation bags that kept their loved ones alive.

The situation was even more unpleasant for the family members of those who died. The three additional volunteers that arrived from the area churches dealt with the suffering of more than a thousand, but there was little information available about how this terrible thing had occurred.

As Raines surveyed the overwhelming surroundings, a tall, graying man in a Philadelphia Fire Department helmet, accompanied by a thin, but elegantly coiffed young blond man, pushed their way into the doctor's progressively smaller area of care.

"I'm Captain Randall Krause," the fireman confidently introduced, "your incident scene commander. This is Frank Slidell, who runs the Philadelphia Federal Emergency Management office. We're about to clear working areas both here and at University Hospital and are setting up a command and communications trailer against the east wall here at Jefferson. We have people and equipment coming from eight other cities, including a Disaster Medical Assistance Team from New Jersey—DMAT. We are commandeering the Pennsylvania Convention Center to house patients, since we already have more than two hundred who need ventilators. Since you seem to be the most experienced guy in mass casualty here, you are now our incident medical director. What else do ya need right now?"

Raines had never been so glad to hear someone else's plan in his entire life.

"Captain, this looks like Botulism to me," he began, "and based on how rapidly my girlfriend was affected after a shower, there has to be a significant concentration of pure toxin in the water supply. We have people here affected after simply brushing their teeth and six poisoned by the overspray in a carwash. We need to shut off the city's water supply now and set up some sort of decontamination station to wash the poison off the victims."

"And what am I supposed to do with a million and a half people with no water supply?" moaned Slidell.

"Get all the bottled water that FEMA has available and ask for a limited call up of Army Reserve and Guard personnel," Raines said. "The Reserve has water purification teams that use reverse osmosis units to make clean water. They can take raw water directly from the Delaware. The National Guard has civil assistance teams trained in dealing with weapons of mass destruction. They can bring decontamination equipment, testing resources, and treatment personnel."

"So how do we go about doing the decontamination until the cavalry arrives?" asked Krause.

"Start with five-gallon sprayers with bleach-and-water solution, then rinse them with hoses. The runoff water will be contaminated, and we need somebody from waste water to advise us on cleaning it up before it goes into the river."

"A U.S. Marine Corps chem-bio unit will have lead elements here within four hours," Krause said. "We're going to have an emergency planning meeting in the command trailer around four o'clock. Join us if you can. Thanks for your suggestions, Doc."

"I'll guess I'll have to make a statement to the press," offered Slidell.

The two civil leaders walked briskly toward the hospital, with Frank Slidell still shaking his head.

~

Huynh Nguyen, a sixty-year-old Vietnamese refugee, stood apart from the crowd, tears streaking his leathery face and collecting on his sparse chin hairs. His words were unintelligible to the paramedic he questioned.

"He wants to know why they died from eating the rice," translated his teenage neighbor.

A man who had survived years of war, escaped from a Southeast Asian country at night in a leaky boat, and traveled across the globe for the simple right to remain alive ... deserved an adequate answer. This man, who dutifully showed up for his school janitorial job each morning, needed to know why his mother, wife, and children had been taken away. Three generations of survival despite hardship had been snuffed out by a single family rice bowl.

"I'm so sorry," the paramedic spoke into the tortured man's eyes. "The doctor thinks that the city has been attacked by poison, and there was nothing we could do to help them."

Around eleven a.m., Raines looked up to see Dr. Chris Richards standing at the inner edge of his circle. He looked contemplative and hesitant to approach. Chris was the youngest attending physician on Jefferson's emergency department staff, but he had never been shy or hesitant to handle the tough cases.

"What's up, Chris?" Raines asked as he watched Richards review the details of his shoes.

"I came to relieve you," was Richards's quiet answer. "Matt Kindred needs to see you."

Raines studied the younger man's face, but it revealed no secrets.

"Where is he?" asked Ron.

"In the family conference room," returned the bone-chilling reply from Richards.

"Aimee? ...Is there a problem with Aimee?" moaned Raines, knowing that his partner would not be holding a conference at a time like this for any other reason.

"Yes ... I'm very sorry."

Raines felt a sudden rush of blood to his face and a wave of nausea as he thought of Aimee, dying alone when he should have been there for her.

Chapter 15

THE CALVARY

Destination Philadelphia; 11 September 2008

D r. Al Marshall sank into the vinyl-padded pseudo luxury of the gate at Atlanta's Hartsfield-Jackson International Airport. Marshall was a sophisticated ebony man; tall, yet not as muscular as during the previous year. He wore wire-rimmed glasses and carried a worn computer case. As he clicked open his laptop case, he reflected on all the changes in medicine over just one brief century. His "black bag" was electronic, and his capacity to function depended more on the WiFi connections available than any skill with his hands. His ability to interface with the Centers for Disease Control mainframe was the primary tool that differentiated him from any other infectious disease warrior in the trenches.

He had always thought there would be benefits to climbing the hierarchical ladder in the world's most advanced medical

organization, but even in CDC's number-four leadership
spot, he flew coach. He had not grown up expecting elegance
in poor Eutaw, Alabama—particularly on a tobacco farm
owned by someone else's family in far away Kentucky. His
childhood did not include a private school or a trust fund,
but he had received tools that were more valuable: honesty,
the ability to work long hours without complaint, and a thirst
for knowledge that propelled him into the world of books.
He thought it just bad luck that his childhood had not also
provided him the tools to succeed in a marriage.

This trip was different from earlier ones. This was not
the random selection of a naturally occurring Ebola virus
ravaging a primitive society in West Africa. This was the
willful release of a biologic agent in an American city with
intent to kill, and the intent had been successful: the agent
had affected the lives of thousands in Philadelphia. The goal
was to find the proper antitoxin-and-antibiotic combination
to maximize the number of people still alive tomorrow. He
looked at the time on the Compaq's screen and longed for
the whine of reversing engines that he would hear as the
airliner backed from the gate.

~

Deep in the Jefferson University Hospital morgue, Navy
Captain Tony Mateo scrubbed the cotton-tipped swab inside
the mouth of the fourth corpse, who had most recently been
a Philadelphia restaurant owner. The restaurateur's face
was bloated and blue, and his once-bright green eyes were
frosted with the haze of demise. Mateo carefully applied the
oral sample to the SMART membrane with his gloved hands
and handed the plastic casing to his young commander,
Major Brad Tower.

The SMART membrane was the apex of immunologic
diagnostic technology. Although only two inches square, the
slide housed the specific antibodies to dangerous bacteria in

a polymer gel and linked those tools of recognition to color-producing enzymes. The enzyme-linked, or ELISA-based, slide simply turned purple when it was touched with the antigens of dangerous bacteria. This particular slide was useful for detecting the presence of the toxin from *Clostridium botulinum* germs.

Mateo was old by military standards—just over sixty—but his square jaw and gray crew cut still broadcast the competence he had gained in more than thirty-five years in navy medicine. He had arrived at the enviable position in life where he no longer had to care if someone didn't like the things he said. He had known the CNO, the Chief of Naval Operations, as a fresh butter-bar ensign and had earned the capacity to speak frankly.

Mateo turned back to the businessman's body and obtained a second oral swab, which he immersed in a broth solution for the polymerase chain reaction search for the offending bacteria to be carried out after arrival of the unit's full diagnostic power. The PCR studies would be able to magnify even minute bits of bacterial DNA to maximize the pick-up of the germ.

"It's the same as the others," announced Marine Corps Major Tower through the thin plastic of his biologic containment suit. "High concentrations of botulinum toxin A in the mouth and on the hands but none on other body surfaces."

Muscular and sandy-haired, Tower was thirty-three and served as the acting commander of the U.S. Marine Chemical and Biologic Incident Response Force. The last three of his fourteen years in the Marines had been filled with planning for a national response to an unprecedented catastrophe such as this.

The two military officers had flown in by commercial air from their base in Indian Head, Maryland within four hours of their call from the Marine 2nd Expeditionary Unit. The trip to Philadelphia was only eventful for the toothpaste.

The two CBIRF leaders had driven up I-295 from Maryland to Washington's Reagan International Airport. They entered the airport security checkpoint, and Tower as usual, presented the TSA agent his active-duty Marine Corps ID and his orders authorizing travel with his assigned personal weapon. The TSA Supervisor was then summoned, and a through search of his briefcase carried out. The senior agent paid little attention to the M-9 Berretta pistol, but seemed concerned about the size of the toothpaste tube in Tower's shaving kit. The problem was resolved when Tower simply suggested the security force discard the toothpaste to remove any risks to the flight.

The military men had arrived in Philadelphia at 1500 hours, placing Tower's deadline for the operational planning of the mission less than four hours away. After the preparations by their advance team leaders, the remainder of their 280-man unit would arrive via a C-5 Galaxy transport aircraft at 2200 hours.

After three years of working together in five different countries, the two officers had settled into a comfortable father/son-style relationship, with Tower always mindful of the military courtesy due to the senior, O-6 grade physician. In the more than four dozen prior deployments of the CBIRF, the goal had been training. This was their initial call for an exposure to a real biologic agent that left real people dying.

Captain Mateo looked at his watch and the broth samples in his aluminum briefcase.

"If we hurry, we can get a preliminary bacterial read before the command meeting at four."

The two military officers retreated to the two cases of equipment that they had spread on the morgue's reception desk, with Tower allowing the senior officer to walk in front of him. Mateo removed the first set of swabs from the broth and touched each to a rapid antigen slide test for Clostridium bacteria, adding tests for anthrax and plague, just for the purposes of having negative controls. In two minutes, the colorimetric indicators on the plastic casing indicated a negative result for each germ. Mateo repeated the testing with samples from the other three deceased patients and found the germ identification results to be consistent, and only the traces of a Botulinum toxin found.

"Don't really understand this," remarked the captain. "How the hell did they get high concentrations of botulinum toxin with absolutely no Clostridial germs present?"

"I guess their players are getting to be a bit more scientifically advanced," said Tower. "The FEMA guy said that he called in the epidemic investigation team from the CDC. They must be sending in a 'germ guy.'"

"We'll confirm these negatives with the polymerase chain equipment when it gets here," shrugged Mateo. "But I'll bet ya a beer that we ain't gonna find no Clostridium germs!"

"I don't understand, Captain," puzzled Tower. "What is the advantage of an attack striking a target with the bacteria filtered out of the toxin mix?"

"Beats me, Brad," Mateo said. "But there's got to be some biologic advantage here that we just don't see yet. Let's get to the meeting."

Chapter 16

FAITHFUL FLIGHT

Destination Texas; 11–12 September 2008

Dr. Ali Zarif clicked off CNN with mixed emotions. The early reports indicated there were over a thousand victims of a toxic or poison exposure in Philadelphia, with the nature of the agent yet to be determined. However, there was also a report of gunfire and arrests in an isolated park near Yonkers, New York. Most importantly, the early reports did not indicate that the water supply was suspect or instruct the citizens to avoid it.

Allah's work goes well, at least in Philadelphia, he thought. *Fear and confusion will build until the Great Satan falls to its knees.*

He reached for the encrypted cell phone on his desk and dialed the number from memory.

"The early reports are favorable," he said in Arabic, with conscious decision to avoid mentioning the fiasco in New

York. "What is your progress?"

Ahmed Madawi nodded with a sigh of thankfulness at the information.

"We are between Knoxville and Birmingham," Madawi said, "and expect to be at our destination by morning prayers. What of Musa?"

"He will sleep with the container, *Ishna' Allah.*" instructed Zarif.

"So it shall be, Teacher," dutiful young follower responded.

Zarif picked up his briefcase and planned to be early for his eleven o'clock class.

~

The National Security Agency's senior analyst for domestic intercepts looked at the Cray supercomputer's screen and the three cell phone calls of interest placed over the last hours. His screening terms were "Philadelphia" and "Allah," and the search included calls made or received within a five-hundred-mile radius of Philadelphia. Two of the calls were in English and the text seemed innocent enough, but the computer identified the third call's language to be Arabic.

The analyst picked up the phone and dialed the number for NSA linguistics.

"Morning, guys," he said. "You got an Arabic speaker there this morning? Great—I'm sending the file now."

~

Just after eight a.m. on September 12, the worn blue International truck, with its container that both caused and carried death, pulled into the gates of the Paris Dredging Company in Texas City, Texas. The three young men in the cab saw buildings made of rusting tin and dirty brown blocks, two aging cranes, and only a few disinterested workers. A rusting metal pier jutted into the brown waters of the industrial canal, which in turn led through the south basin to the Texas City harbor.

On the water's surface at the pier languished an ancient working barge, a curious concoction of a flat metal deck, several non-working generators, two sometimes-working welding machines, and a well-worn crane that hovered like a hulking dinosaur. Without words of welcome, the crane operator motioned the truck forward and then signaled for the passengers to clear the area.

After more than forty years of operating cranes on the waterfront, Hollis Rampart no longer asked questions. His paunch was not quite as tight in his overalls as it had been during 2007, and his bank statement was an absolute embarrassment. The dredging company had seen boom times and bust, and Rampart only wanted to funnel enough cash into the decrepit company to keep the bank off his back. The addition of the casinos to the Texas Gulf coast had been the final straw financially, and just last week he had lost enough money to pay another miserly payroll.

"I don't care what they want me to dump in the Gulf," he told himself, "as long as it's heavy enough to stay on the bottom."

For this job, he had eight tons of concrete rejects for ballast and a location three miles offshore, where artificial reef material would not seem out of place. The arrangements would give him fifteen thousand dollars and a truck to sell, just for two days of work and the ability to keep his mouth shut.

As the boom of the crane swung over the truck, the three Faithful walked through the dredge company's front gate and down the cracked sidewalk that ran by the potholed street.

The map indicated that it was just over a mile to the rental car agency.

~

At four p.m., Ahmed Madawi drove the rented Impala, as Mohammed and Farouk slept in the rear. The light brown sedan slowed and turned into the parking lot of the Bilal Islamic Center of Houston, Texas.

The five million citizens of the Space City metropolitan area did not notice the new arrivals to the city. The oil refineries and rubber plants, banking headquarters and medical research centers continued an uninterrupted buzz of weekday activity.

Only the Islamic Center noticed the arrival of the three young Arabic men.

Imam Hafiz met the young men as they removed their shoes and entered the place of worship.

"Welcome, young travelers," Hafiz beamed. "Dr. Zarif has e-mailed that you will be with us for a time, and of your plans to continue your studies here."

The three young men did not respond, since they were unsure if the imam had any information on their recent activities.

"He tells me that you are among the most faithful and will be special tools of Allah," added the imam.

When it was apparent that the religious leader knew them only as travelers and students, they began to relax and listen to the plans for their housing and support.

"We are grateful for the hospitality of our Brothers," smiled Madawi, "and will be of service to you in all tasks."

"We would like to hear of your travels and service to Allah," Imam Hafiz requested, "after Friday prayers."

The imam led the two Faithful to a small, dormitory-style room containing bunk beds, prayer rugs, and several copies of the Qur'an. They were encouraged to use the mosque's kitchen and the computer terminal in the Bilal Center's office.

After the imam departed, Madawi typed out a brief message to the encrypted mailbox of Dr. Zarif, confirming their safe arrival and readiness to further the work of Allah. Mohammed turned on the satellite television monitor in the community center and found the channel already tuned to Al-Jezeera.

The story being broadcast showed footage of the hundreds of the toxin affected lying on the sidewalks and parking lots of Philadelphia's Jefferson and University hospitals. After a brief discussion of the source of the toxic assault—still unknown—the footage showed hundreds of people walking in a Philadelphia shopping mall with no ill effects from the attack.

"Allah has spoken to the people of America," commented a bearded young student from Kuwait.

"We expected many more to fall to the sword of Allah," Mohammed spoke quietly.

"For the sword to fall upon a thousand unbelievers is well worth our sacrifice," Madawi reassured him. "remember that Dr. Zarif tells us that the blessing has not yet completed its work. On the third day, the Shari'a of Allah will be made clear to the unbelievers."

Chapter 17

INCIDENT COMMAND

Philadelphia; 11 September 2008

D r. Ron Raines had been up for twenty-six hours when he remembered the four o'clock meeting of the people who would deal with the nation's greatest tragedy. Eight doctors now covered the Jefferson ER, and more than two dozen paramedics were working the crowds to select the most acutely ill. As he left his position in the parking lot, Raines was astounded at the war zone–like appearance around the hospital.

Vehicles, many with doors hanging open, choked the streets in the positions that their owners had left them. A tangle of ambulances remained near the entrance bay and paper littered the sidewalks. Hundreds of people had already been ferried to the Pennsylvania Convention Center, although Raines had no idea who was caring for them in their new location.

Raines found the trailer at ten minutes after four and heard the controversy that erupted through the thin aluminum walls. The trailer was rusting, dented, and had been attached recently to a temporary power pole.

Raines climbed the steps into a scene of near chaos. The two dozen folding chairs in the center of the trailer were packed, and the surrounding walls were stacked two and three deep with people attempting to ask questions. Captain Krause stood near a desk on the right wall of the command trailer, repeatedly trying to get the group's attention. The room's inhabitants talked loudly their attempts to explain the event, and Raines overheard the words "Russians" and "military nerve gas" and "PCB's."

"Let's get started …" Krause began. The droning of many voices with little actual knowledge continued.

The fire captain stepped into an adjacent storeroom and returned with a battery-operated bullhorn.

"Let's get started!" Krause repeated as the echo of his electronically enhanced voice commanded the attention of the crowd. He motioned for silence.

Randall Krause was in his late forties, handsome, with graying dark hair and the remnants of a muscular build. As a veteran of a lifelong career a Philadelphia city fireman, Krause felt that his ragged old Bronco and cheap shoes branded him as a career firefighter; but the boys at the station knew that his two divorces and the big, stainless-steel chronometer watch really marked him as a "fully qualified" fireman. Over the last eighteen years, his responsibility for his "boys" had extended to the occupants of four stationhouses.

He had spent years training for any event that might threaten the survival of his city, but he never thought he would put this training into action. On his desk sat a bulging three-ring binder with the names and phone numbers of the resources he was now contacting for the first time.

Placing the bullhorn onto the desk in front of him, the fireman asserted his leadership of the assembled group.

"I'm Captain Randall Krause," he began, "your incident commander and the man you should contact with your needs and suggestions, at any time of the day or night. Obviously, we are involved in a catastrophe of historic proportions, and I have asked each of you here as representatives of organizations needed to help our citizens survive. I am contacting every resource I can find. We have to limit the progression of this horrible thing, coordinate our care efforts, and direct the population into activities that will accomplish something. I'm going to introduce a few of you and request you tell us your progress thus far. Mr. Slidell?"

The man who stood in response to Krause was thirty, with carefully sprayed blonde hair and blue contact lenses. His precise diction was one indication that he preferred acting to politics. His acting income, however, was low enough that he required the steady income of a bureaucrat to pay rent on his Society Hill apartment.

"I am Frank Slidell," the man announced from his position in the spotlight. "I am the local director of the Federal Emergency Management Agency and will be responsible for the coordination of federal reactions to this crisis. We have announced to the public that the city has suffered an attack with an unknown toxin, possibly as a 9/11 terrorist anniversary event. Based on Dr. Raines's recommendation, we have closed the city's water supply and have requested the mobilization of an Army Reserve water purification detachment. Citizens will be required to use only bottled water until the reverse osmosis purification units are online. We have requested that the governor declare Philadelphia a disaster area and mobilize civil support/weapons of mass destruction units from the National Guard.

"We have activated our national medical disaster system," Slidell droned on, "and have requested the mobilization of the NJ-1 Disaster Medical Assistance Team from New Jersey to assist with the care of the ill that we have started delivering to the Pennsylvania Convention Center. We anticipate the DMAT's arrival tomorrow morning. I will handle all of the public relations and would appreciate your offices referring the press to my office."

"Thank you, Frank," Captain Krause cut in.

Slidell sat down with an air of frustration. It was not easy for Slidell to play the game of fitting in; particularly when the local officials were buffoons and the sluggish remnants of a culture that ended decades before. His importance in this event was not yet appreciated.

"Ms. Graves?" Krause called next.

A pretty woman with short dark hair and a plain business suit that hugged her frame, struggled to stand near the center of the room.

"I'm Melissa Graves of the Red Cross," she said quietly. "We will assist with food and communication in an area of the Crisis Center being set up within the Convention Center. We will attempt to maintain a database of those ill and deceased and communicate with family members who contact the city for information. We will undoubtedly need funds far in excess of our budget to respond to this catastrophe."

Graves sat heavily, the needs of the city and the funding for those needs swirling in her mind. Over the last two years, her world had revolved around her ongoing divorce and the needs of her son, but now the stark reality of the measures needed for the city's survival was staggering.

Dr. Raines was Krause's next choice, surprising Ron with his prominent position in the introductions. Raines stood and wondered if he looked as rough as he felt.

"I am Dr. Ron Raines," he began. "I am representing Jefferson University Hospital's emergency department, and I guess I'm now the medical director this ordeal. I have a military background that may be helpful in recognizing the biowarfare agents that have been directed against us. Of course, no one can now be sure, but from a military medicine point of view, some things are clear at this stage. This is some type of toxin, and the majority of people we have seen were contaminated through the city water supply. We have seen people affected by showers, by a car wash, and even by just brushing their teeth.

"The contamination had to come in after the water went through the treatment plants," Raines continued, "or the plants' processing would have removed it. This toxin acts a little like an organophosphate poison, with paralysis and respiratory failure, but we are not seeing seizures or excessive lung and airway secretions, as we would with a nerve agent. I suspect that we are dealing with botulinum toxin."

"And we have confirmed those suspicions," added the arthritic, gray-haired man who wore a neatly pressed Navy battle dress uniform.

"Please continue, Captain," Krause requested of the man.

"I'm Tony Mateo of the Marine Corps Chem-Bio Incident Response Force, and this young officer is my commander, Major Brad Tower."

Raines, and a few others with military pasts, noted the polished silver eagles and the surface warfare badge on the older man's BDUs. The muscular young major's chest displayed impressive Recon Marine wings, and he wore a pistol belt and sidearm.

"Our Marine unit is trained to deal with national emergencies such as this, but our treatment capabilities are limited to numbers in the hundreds," reported Captain Mateo. "We have confirmed high concentrations of botulinum toxin on the hands and in the mouths of several of the deceased, which is damn worrisome, since it only takes a spot of pure toxin the size of the dot over an 'i' to kill eight to ten adult humans. In our preliminary tests," he continued, "we've been unable to find any of the Clostridium germs that produce the toxin. We understood that perhaps someone would be here from the CDC—"

"That's me," said a thin, black man wearing wire-rimmed glasses and a casual tan windbreaker. "I'm Dr.Al Marshall, an infectious disease consultant with the Centers for Disease Control. I really can't explain why the ELISA tests do not show the germ as well as the toxin, but would suggest that we place all of the affected individuals on empiric antibiotic coverage for *Clostridium botulinum.* As for the botulinum toxin," Marshall continued, "we should concentrate our care on supportive measures and using a specific antiserum. We have the SNS, a strategic national stock of antibiotics, antitoxins, and even ventilators to access, and we should be able to get the initial deliveries of the medical equipment here by morning. We'll have the Pennsylvania State Lab in Pittsburgh do full cultures of the oral cavity, blood, and urine of several of the deceased patients to try to isolate the organism."

"Botulinum toxin can be inactivated by heat and by low pH," added Marshall, "so flushing the city's water supply with dilute hydrochloric acid will hopefully clear the toxin from the lines. FEMA should encourage Philadelphians to use boiled water to clean dishes and silverware."

"Emergency medical services?" called Krause when Marshall had finished.

A white-hired man in an EMS uniform stepped forward and reported assets from twelve other counties working in Philadelphia and senior paramedics providing triage at Jefferson, University, and Hahnemann hospitals. He told of beginning the transports of toxin-affected patients to the Convention Center, but finding only a few volunteers there to care for the patients. He begged for doctors and nurses to be there for the seriously ill that would be transported before the DMAT's arrival."

Krause furiously scribbled his thoughts on a television announcement to try to obtain medical personnel, while FEMA director Slidell just nodded dumbly.

"Law enforcement?" Krause asked next.

Two of the suited men standing near the trailer's back wall gave almost imperceptible nods. The older of the two wore a dark blue suit, and his steel-gray hair was cut short in military style. As he spoke, he nodded toward a young man nearby who was a bit overdressed for a catastrophe.

"I'm Special Agent Landrum, and this is Special Agent Deason," noted the gray-haired suit, "from the FBI's Philadelphia field office."

Krause and the group waited for further comment, and expected at least a limited briefing on suspect organizations that might have been behind the attack. When the FBI agents offered nothing more than their names, Krause put them in the limelight in his normally blunt fashion.

"Okay, what do ya know so far?" he asked.

With the typical hedging of a man with a legal degree, young Deason began with "We're not at liberty—" only to be cut short by a blast from a furious fire captain.

"Your liberty, my ass!" exploded Krause. "You can put away the rulebook, young man, because if any lives are to be saved, it will be by the people in this room."

Deason looked at Landrum and said quietly, "We'll have to clear release of ongoing investigation information with our headquarters."

"Fine," retorted Krause. "In the meantime, you can clear the hell out of my meeting!"

The FBI suits slunk from the room, leaving a third man, with a much more rumbled appearance, remaining in the background. The man was of average height and build, somewhere in his fifties, and much less flashy than the FBI agents. Krause could just discern traces of a wry smile beginning at the corners of his mouth.

"And you, sir?" Krause demanded of the man, angry daggers still visible in his dark eyes.

The fiftyish man in the rumpled brown suit spoke with

quiet confidence.

"Talbot ... National Security," he said simply.

"From ...the White House?" questioned Krause in confusion.

"No, OGA," Talbot responded. "And I don't believe in rulebooks."

Although only a few in the crowd understood "OGA," Raines had firsthand knowledge of the term from his Ranger years, and the Marines in the room smiled. Tower and Mateo worked with "other governmental agencies" on almost all of their operations. Whether Talbot was from CIA or NSA was not important, he would be just as unlikely to discuss who signed his paycheck.

"Early this morning," the rumpled man divulged, "unknown assailants entered the Philadelphia Water Department's Pumping Station A, the first in a series of pressure stations to pump clean water after it exits the Baxter Purification Plant. Three workmen and a guard were killed at the station, and an eighteen-wheeler was backed into the facility. This is the suspected entry point for the water supply contamination. We are told that the pumping station has direct or indirect ties to all of the water lines feeding northern Philadelphia."

"Damn!" Krause exploded. "That's gotta be more than three-quarters of a million people!"

"Eight hundred and forty thousand is the number we calculated," reported Talbot gravely.

～

The line of very worried professionals filed down the steps of the trailer to the parking lot amid yells of "Do you have a statement?" and "Kelly Crockett, Action Six News! Could we have a comment, please?"

A subtly smiling Slidell held court for the glaring lights of the six cameramen and gave party line answers to the reporters' questions.

Ron Raines smiled as he heard the would-be actor hamming up his national exposure with comments of a "heinous attack" by "ruthless terrorists" bent on "destruction of our American way of life." He did at least give the public information on the danger of the water supply and the importance of boiling eating utensils, and he suggested than any ill persons report to Jefferson Hospital, University Hospital, or the Pennsylvania Convention Center.

A star is born! thought Raines.

Chapter 18

TRUCKS

Philadelphia; 11 September 2008

After leaving the incident command meeting, Ron Raines walked with leaden feet toward Jefferson University Hospital's basement morgue. With a determined sigh, he pushed open the double doors and entered the brightly lit room, now filled to overflowing with the stretchers of the dead. At the desk by the entrance, Raines saw a young pathology tech in a stained lab coat listening to blues music and eating a sandwich.

"Hey," Raines greeted him with the words that he wished to God were not true: "I lost someone earlier today, and I'd like to see her."

"Sorry for that, Doc," replied the young man. "What was her name?"

"Aimee. Aimee Hargrove," Raines told him. "Around

eleven this morning."

The blues fan looked through a sheaf of papers and then shook his head. "I purely lost track of all the names when it got so busy," he said, "but she ain't in here. She'd have to be outside."

"Outside?" Raines asked, puzzled.

"Yeah," the young man reported, "the FEMA guys got two refrigerated tractor-trailer rigs for all the bodies, but you ain't ever gonna find her."

"Why not?" asked the doctor, long used to overcoming obstacles.

"See for y'sef," the young man said as he pointed to the corridor and the exit sign at its end.

Raines, short on patience and long on fatigue, finished the journey down the hall and exited onto the hospital's rear loading dock. He saw four men in surgical gowns and masks loading body bags into the rear of the tractor-trailer rigs backed up to the dock. A guard with a familiar face supervised the loading and wrote down the toe-tag names on a clipboard.

"Hey, Dr. R," said the guard. "What are you doing way down here?"

"It's my girlfriend," Raines stated solemnly. "She died around eleven this morning."

"Gee, I'm sorry, Doc," the guard said with real understanding in his voice, "but we aren't going to be able to find her for several days."

After seeing Raines's perplexed look, he pointed into the back of the truck. The body bags were stacked like human firewood, a dozen wide and eight to ten bodies high. Lifeless elbows prodded into equally lifeless necks and faces. Over half of the forty-foot-long trailer was already packed with the people who awoke that morning to go to jobs, to visit family members, or to walk in the Historic District—to simply begin the next day of the lives that they had been given. They had no warning that by afternoon, they would be stacked in the back of a truck, their only remaining connection to the lives they once lived a handwritten tag on their right big toes.

Ron Raines was exhausted as he climbed the stairs to the emergency department. Although he knew he would function better after a brief nap before beginning a new shift, he did not think he would be able to sleep. Not only was he worried about the critically ill but untreated, who might still be left in the crowds, he felt crippling guilt for leaving Aimee in her hour of greatest need. In addition, he still faced an unpleasant task.

Ron slipped into the Jefferson ER call room, sat at the desk, and stared at the telephone on its surface. He lifted the receiver and then returned it to the cradle. It was only five p.m. in Boston, and it would be difficult to find Aimee's parents during the rush hour.

They may have heard about the attack on CNN. They need to know now, not later, thought Raines, as he attempted to lift the receiver again. Now he believed the description that he had heard from suicidal people who most needed to make calls for help: the receiver seemed to weigh five hundred pounds.

Well, it's just like jump school, he thought. *Time to "stand in the door."*

With this final bit of determination, he dialed Mr. Hargrove's cell number.

"Yes…" answered the older man in a strained voice.

"Its Ron," Raines began slowly. "I'm afraid that I must give you horrible news. There has been a biological attack in north Philadelphia, apparently with a toxin distributed through the water supply. Aimee was exposed to the agent while taking a shower, and then had paralysis and difficulty breathing." The clinician in Raines knew he should use the words "dead," not "passed away" or "expired." His training taught him that people could easily misunderstand these words that did not hit them bluntly between the eyes, yet it just seemed cruel to say the words "dead" to the father of an only daughter.

"Is she alive?" was the simple question from Hargrove.

"No, and I'm so sorry..." said Raines. "Despite all the hospital could do..."

There was a long silence from the phone in Boston.

"I'm sure you did whatever you could," replied Hargrove flatly, though Raines imagined that his thoughts continued: "but you didn't save her."

"I can't possibly understand how you feel," were the words that found their way to Raines's mouth, "but I'm hurting, too." It would simply be insulting to tell this man that he could understand his pain in losing Aimee.

"Things are a mess here," said Raines. "I have no idea how quickly funerals will even be possible."

"Thank you for the call," choked Hargrove, as he pressed the "End" button on the cell.

"How can things get so bad in such short time?" Raines wondered aloud, but heard no answers. He curled onto the call bed and covered his head with a pillow.

~

"Yes, sir," Randall Krause begged the FoodLand manager, "if there is any possible way. We already have a trailer and a half loaded and will need at least two more ... Yes, in the morning will be fine ... Thank you, sir." Krause banged the phone into the cradle more loudly than he desired.

"What kinds of crazies kill innocent women and children?" he asked the incident command firemen who overheard his request for more refrigerated trailers. "I've been in this town for more than thirty years, and I just don't understand it. Surely God has a special place in hell for this level of evil."

Chapter 19

DMAT/DMORT

New Jersey; 12 September 2008

D r. Jillian Case watched the expansion gaps in the concrete highway flash by her passenger-side bus window. The convoy streaked southwest on the New Jersey Turnpike, and their destination was very likely the worst disaster to ever befall an American city. Her caravan of four tractor-trailer rigs and two buses departed Trenton, New Jersey on the morning of September 12 for the brief three-hour drive to the besieged city.

The preparations for the deployment of NJ-1 were anything but brief. The team had been in existence since 1990, formed from the plans initiated by the U.S. Public Health Service through its newly conceived National Disaster Medical System. The team had evolved through extensive training, hurricane deployments, and personnel changes and now was one of the nation's most experienced level one disaster medical assistance teams. Over three million dollars worth of federally funded medical equipment and supplies had been carefully maintained by the fire/rescue, medical, nursing, and EMT members of NJ-1, and their monthly training sessions were well attended by the civic-minded group of professionals.

As the team leader, Jillian Case volunteered to back burner her family medicine teaching job at Robert Wood Johnson Medical School for two days each month; then spend hundreds of hours planning for the team's deployment when the unit was needed. The young doctor—petite, blonde, and quiet—had driven to Trenton from New Brunswick on the afternoon of the disaster to ready the team for departure. Providing patient care to the seriously ill in the DMAT tents and the Philadelphia Convention Center would be vastly different than her normal job of supervising residents in a modern hospital facility.

John Harrell, the DMAT's senior nurse, had also started his personal involvement early. He was the director of the emergency department at the university's affiliate, Cooper Hospital in Camden, only eight miles from the Philadelphia disaster. He arranged for Cooper's ambulances and off-duty-staff assistance on the morning of the Philadelphia catastrophe and then drove north to Trenton to gather a full panel of the team's nursing personnel for the NJ-1 deployment. He had prepared Cooper for a two-week absence of the nurses he was stealing.

Gary Schell, the DMAT's senior paramedic, was also from Camden. He joined Harrell as he approached his petite team leader at the rear of the bus.

"You look worried, Doc," said Harrell to Case, his weight-lifter-size body always in contrast with his typically quiet and caring words.

"Nobody's ever done this, John," she sighed. "When we covered Hurricane Katrina, we saw just a few hundred injured, and then all we needed to do was provide convenience care until the power came back up. No team has dealt with hundreds of dead and dying. I'm not worried about those suffering from botulism; we'll either be able to help them or we won't. I'm more concerned about the family members who don't understand what the hell is happening and that everything possible is being done!"

The image of a mob of frightened people storming the triage tent played vividly in Harrell's mind. As Cooper's emergency director, he had lived through scenes of terrified families, out of control following a traumatic death—but not those same awful tensions multiplied by the thousands.

Gary Schell, graying and stretching the seams of his worn coveralls, sat by the tiny doctor and smiled. After navigating more than twenty-five years of street life as a paramedic for Camden fire and rescue, his duties were now more often making schedules than providing patient care—but his hide was ironclad.

"We'll handle it fine, Doc," Schell reassured Case. "I'll make commo with the Philly PD when we arrive and set up a police security team for each shift. If anything, we've got more people and resources than we've ever taken into a situation."

"You have John to thank for that," nodded Case. "I guess people will do anything to get out of a hospital for a few days."

The Disaster Medical Assistance Team's staffing was unusual in its addition of two pharmacists for the management of inpatient or outpatient medications, and even three social workers for assistance with emergency funds, emergency childcare, and contacting distant family members who needed information on the welfare of their loved ones in the disaster area.

"I'm not sure how many of the Mortuary Assistance Team members are coming from their base in South Carolina," Dr. Case added, "but the team leader is a man named Palmer

Grace, a forensic dental surgeon from Charleston. The team will identify the dead by eyewitnesses and dental records, mostly, but they even have two forensic pathologists able to use DNA techniques if we have no clues as to someone's identity.

"They have the military field version of Canon's latest digital x-ray equipment for rapid dental record matching," she continued. "The setup uses a laptop computer rather than film so that they can send a set of digital images by telephone modem to any dental office that holds an old set of x-rays. They even have a team of volunteers from the Funeral Directors Association to do emergency embalming. The FEMA people on the scene tell me that they already have a refrigeration truck loaded with bodies."

"Nothing is going to make this situation nice," admitted Harrell, "but we can make it better than if we had stayed home."

As Dr. Case stared out of the bus's tinted window, her blue eyes took in the auto salvage yards, paving contractors, metal fabricators and distribution warehouses, the sagging power lines and unending miles of highway. *Garden State, indeed*, she thought.

∼

Frank Slidell and the Philadelphia police had barricaded off the western half of the Convention Center parking lot for the use of the DMAT's triage and treatment tents. As the group of medical personnel began to unload the IV fluids, defibrillators, and gurneys, Jill Case noted the approach of a carefully coiffed Slidell, walking with a distinguished, white-haired man who was wearing outdated platinum-rimmed eyeglasses and a well-worn gray suit.

"Dr. Case, this is Dr. Palmer Grace, the team leader for the Disaster Mortuary Assistance Team," announced Slidell with theatrical enunciation.

"It is a great pleasure to meet you, Dr. Case," said Dr. Grace. Case thought he seemed quite polished for a man whose conversational skills must have been honed while looking at the teeth of the dead.

"Please call me Jill," smiled Case, liking the sophisticated old dental surgeon immediately. "And please let me know if any of the resources of our DMAT can be of assistance to you."

"We are completing our setup and will be based in the Jefferson University Hospital morgue," offered Grace. "We are self-sufficient, but of course, such a deluge of death is an unknown experience in the United States."

"Our living accommodations are a bit spartan," said Jill almost apologetically, "however, we're quite sociable. We're setting up our sleep tents behind the treatment area and will be ready to start triaging patients around six this evening."

～

John Harrell placed the triage log book on a collapsible table by the tent's entrance. As he reviewed the otoscopes, IV catheters, and rolls of tape, he thought of his daughter. She was not like other fourteen-year-old girls, and she worried when he was gone for even a few days. He had always been her protector, particularly through the dark days of her heart surgery when she was four. Today, she had stood at the door as he left; anxiously rubbing her nose and repeatedly pushing her glasses back up into place. She was bright for a child with Down syndrome and sensitive to the feelings of her family members.

I'll call her before we get too busy, Harrell promised himself.

Gary Schell had not sweated this much in years. After raising the three tents, he and his medics began to string up rope walkways to guide patients into the triage area. His senior paramedics would triage patients with the backup of a single doctor as the DMAT nurses assisted with the patients admitted to the Crisis Center. He thought back to his rather unpleasant discussion of the deployment with his Camden fire captain yesterday afternoon, before the team's departure.

"Hell, Gary," griped the captain. "I'm all for helping the needy, but you're taking almost half of my paramedics. What's the city going to do for emergency care?"

"It's only two weeks, Cap!" Schell rationalized. "You know we gotta be where we're needed."

This afternoon, he was carrying an oxygen bottles under each arm when he first felt the discomfort. It started as a fist-like pressure between his shoulder blades and then became a dull ache that radiated into the left side of his neck and left arm. He thought his awkward position carrying the bottles had caused him to pull a muscle, but the pain got worse after he placed the bottles in the triage tent. He vision began to blur, and he threw up.

This is friggin' great, he thought. *We got hundreds of people in need of care, and I have to pick this moment to have a heart attack.*

He walked toward John, who was checking medical supplies against a deployment list.

"Hey John," he asked casually, "is the EKG machine up yet?"

"Yeah, but we don't have power y—"

John stopped short after a single glance at his friend.

"Yeah, I'm having a little chest pain."

"When did this start?" asked John sternly after digesting Gary's ashen color and beads of perspiration on his face.

"About fifteen minutes ago," Gary reported quietly. "I don't feel any premature beats, but I'm getting short of breath … I guess I'm going into congestive heart failure."

John helped Gary climb onto a gurney and then started the oxygen that the paramedic had just wrestled into the tent. The senior nurse then put an aspirin and a nitroglycerine tablet beneath Gary's tongue.

John yelled through the tent flaps to a firefighter working

outside.

"I need that generator running—*now!*"

He attached the EKG monitor pads to Gary's chest and waited impatiently for the magic of electricity.

Within three minutes, the trailer-mounted diesel generator rumbled into life, and the overhead lights in the tent blinked into activity. The EKG paper began to scroll across the machine, John's eyes carefully following the telltale squiggles that forecast Gary's future.

"It's an inferior wall myocardial infarction," reported John gravely. "Is the pain any better after the nitro?"

"Not much," replied Gary. "Now what?"

"Now you get a heart cath," answered John Harrell reassuringly. "We just need to find someplace and somebody to do it."

Chapter 20

CRISIS CENTER

Philadelphia; 12 September 2008

Within the cavernous space of the Pennsylvania Convention Center, the facility remained positioned for the convention of investment bankers that had been meeting there when the disaster struck. Dozens of financial balance sheets littered the exhibit hall tables and floors, and the weary calm of post-Wall Street planning still hung in the air when the first ambulance sirens screamed their arrivals. With the resources for patient care still in the planning stages, only three volunteer nurses and a retired radiologist filtered in to assist during the initial hours. Despite all of the attempts to salvage human life at University, Jefferson and Hahnemann, no balance sheet could have tallied the terror of the life-and-death events unfolding for the first families to arrive for Crisis Center care.

The brilliantly lit floor space contrasted with the dark mood of the families huddled within. During the horrid morning hours of the day before, they had been lying on concrete, in the back seats of cars and in ambulances that could not reach the hospital. Foreign instruments and plastic tubes were poked into body orifices faster than the family members could understand, and they slowly realized that this event was not going away and those items meant life. Those tubes and instruments enabled the simple passage of air into lungs and the breathing that they usually took for granted.

Now people at least had a place. There were no comforts, but they were sheltered from the gathering coolness of the night and began to see the few volunteer health professionals who would answer questions if something seemed wrong. They at least had a focal point for their hope, and they accepted their new care environment with ardor. Both the families of the ill and the thinly stretched volunteer healthcare workers saw the arriving Disaster Medical Assistance Team as a group of knights in shining armor.

The full 300-man complement of the U.S. Marine Chemical and Biologic Incident Response Force arrived at the Pennsylvania Convention Center just before eleven at night, and began to assemble their Decontamination Tents with the efficiency of a well-oiled machine. As the Marine chemical specialists staffed the decontamination area, Marine medics set-up tents for immunizations and secured a storage area within the Convention Center. Marine communications specialists installed a tactical satellite communication system and plugged the receiving end of the network into the side of an unmarked white government van. The rear of the nondescript vehicle housed the operations center of the CBIRF, with Mateo and Tower sharing a metal console and very little space for expansion.

The NJ-1 Disaster Medical Assistance Team erected tents for triage and treatment, in addition to a small sleeping tent for the off-duty healthcare providers. Dr. Case and

John Harrell divided the DMAT personnel into two 12-hour shifts to support 24-hour operations. The DMAT night shift manned the triage and treatment areas with nurses and paramedics, then assigned all remaining staff, including a pharmacist and two social workers to assist the patient care in the Crisis Center. Dr. Case also placed herself into duties in the Convention Center, where the worst of the toxin-affected were continuing to arrive. The senior paramedics in the tent could handle the few ill individuals and family members that were arriving in the DMAT triage and treatment area.

~

"The numbers of the dead and ill are reported by the local Federal Emergency Management office to now soar over 1400 in the Philadelphia metro area alone," blared the Action Six News special report. "The attack hails from an unknown source, but the toxic agent is suspected to be botulism, caused by the *Clostridium botulinum* germ. Credible sources indicate that Philadelphia's water supply is the mode of transmission, and FEMA authorities have ordered that Philadelphia city water sources be strictly avoided and only bottled water used until the crisis has been fully evaluated."

The coolly professional young newscaster continued.

"Any individuals who are experiencing muscle weakness should be immediately evaluated at the newly-established Crisis Center, and citizens with difficulty breathing should call 911 for emergency access to care. The Crisis Center is housed by the Pennsylvania Convention Center and can be approached from Arch Street or Race Street here in Philadelphia. Stand by for the latest on the developing events on your trusted news source, Action Six News."

~

The Marines and the DMAT rapidly divided the responsibilities of the Crisis Center care, and the group planned to move into long-term daily function. Dr. Marshall was to be the physician team leader for the twelve-hour day shift, while Captain Mateo was responsible for the night hours. The first night in the Crisis Center, however, did not allow the luxury of rest periods. Drs. Mateo, Marshall and Case all stayed awake caring for Crisis Center patients and talking to distressed family members.

By morning on September 13th, only four of the national strategic stock ventilators that arrived on the previous evening remained in reserve for even more extreme circumstances. Still, the supply of breathing machines was so far short of the patients needing assistance that Ambu bags and the dedicated love of their family members supported over a hundred of the toxin-affected. Major Tower supervised the herding of all of the individuals ill with muscle weakness into the Marine decontamination unit before they were allowed into the DMAT triage and treatment tents. The major balanced the supply needs and wants, and reported the unit's activities to Colonel Steele, the commander of the 4th Marine Expeditionary Unit. Slidell enjoyed his role of official spokesman for the news hungry reporters from more than twenty national press and television outlets.

Despite the hours-long lines, most of the family members were taking advantage of the sandwich and soup stations set up by the Red Cross in the food court on the Center's third floor. Almost all of the families had visited the communication area, where the Convention Center's second floor bank of twenty-four phone lines had been opened for the free Red Cross calls that allowed distraught family members to reassure distant relatives that their loved one was, at least, still alive.

～

As mid-day approached on the sunny morning of September 13, Tower noted that number of people presenting for triage had significantly dropped. He talked with Dr. Case and Marshall and suggested that after a harrowing day and a half, the horror of the attack had reached its peak and that if the new presentations continued to drop, survival of the city just might be possible. Perhaps the combined efforts of the entire team could force the crisis under control, rather than simply turning another page in a nightmare book that no one really wanted to read.

During the shift change briefing at six on the evening of the 13th, Marshall summarized: "At two days into the attack," summarized Dr. Al Marshall on the morning of September 13, "Philadelphia has over 800 dead and more than 900 affected but still alive. Just over 700 of the survivors are here in the Crisis Center, and nearly 200 are under care at Philadelphia hospitals pending transport. We have 247 patients needing ventilatory support, and we are using all of the strategic national stock ventilators available. We are hopeful for more ventilators from federal sources by tomorrow morning, but still have more than a hundred family members breathing for their own loved ones."

Marshall scratched his thatch of dark, curly hair in thought.

"We have completed the administration of two doses of botulinum antitoxin to the patients on respiratory support," the infectious disease doctor said and one to those under observation without an endotracheal tube. We have enough strategic stock antitoxin to last less than twenty-four hours," he said, "but we are expecting a direct shipment from Sanofi-Pasteur, the manufacturer.

"So what you're saying," stated Mateo, "is that we're screwed beyond all belief."

"Yeah," Marshall admitted, "but don't give up the ship. The number of ill sent from area hospitals has drastically decreased during the day, and we are hopeful this thing is ending. We lost only four more patients during the last twelve hours. We're giving intravenous ampicillin to the ventilated people, and oral ciprofloxacin those who are ambulatory, until we get the culture results from the Pennsylvania state lab. If the cultures confirms the CBIRF's findings of this being just toxin and not live germs, we may be able to stop the antibiotic therapy.

"The antitoxin is equine, not a recombinant product?" asked Dr. Mateo.

"Afraid so," Marshall replied. "We haven't had any anaphylactoid reactions yet, but even using skin testing for horse serum allergy before giving the drug, we'll run into some late-onset serum sickness problems."

Marshall tried to remember how long it had been since he had actually tried to resuscitate a patient dying of an allergic reaction. Had it really been twelve years before, while he was in residency? There were a couple of resuscitation attempts during a deployment to Kenya for an Ebola outbreak, but others had taken the lead role in providing the care. He had been responsible for decisions on the treatment protocols, but missed most of the hands-on medicine. He had spent years in administration, but the situation now was up close and personal.

With a hidden smile, Marshall watched his colleague, the grizzled Captain Mateo, stand at the helm of his current ship. Mateo leaned one elbow on a resuscitation crash cart and repeatedly surveyed the patients scattered across the gray-carpeted floors. Marshall trusted that this rough-hewn old doctor would have pushed epinephrine and steroids into a patient with serious allergic problems before he himself could have even opened the crash cart. No experience aside from watching many people die enabled such a degree of comfort under pressure.

"What kind of late problems do you expect from the anti-toxin?" asked Major Tower.

"Mostly rashes and low-grade fever," noted Marshall, "but some will have joint pain, fever, lymph node problems, and recurrent hives for months."

"It's still a small price to pay to be alive and free of a venti-lator," commented Mateo.

Marshall nodded through his fatigue.

"Any questions or comments?" asked Marshall.

No questions followed, and the group stood and began to disperse.

Captain Tony Mateo was the first to stand, and he put his hand on the shoulder of Marshall's green scrub top.

"We really appreciate you taking time away from your family and office to help us out with this one," said Mateo graciously.

The CDC doctor's face looked crestfallen, although Mateo did not know why. Marshall just nodded, but he didn't want to explain himself as he thought of his ex-wife, ex-house, and ex-dog.

"My family is really just a five-year-old daughter," Marshall confided. "She'll be easily bought off with a Liberty Bell souvenir from downtown."

"How about you guys?" Marshall asked. "You're certainly not in uniform for the money."

"You can say that again," laughed Mateo, pulling out and balancing his wallet on his right index fingertip.

"Even though I have to be away from them, I'm here because of my family," admitted Tower. "I've got a pair of sons, and I want them to grow up without all the dangers that I spend my time worrying about. I guess I do it for my dad, too. He was a jarhead and served on Guadalcanal. He never left."

Mateo chimed in. "My old battle-ax wouldn't know what to do with me puttering around the house all the time," he grinned. "After thirty-four years, what's left to talk about?"

"Aw, Captain," argued Tower, "you know you can't stand to be away from that woman."

"Well, I admit she's kinda' grown on me," Mateo smiled.

"I got a daughter in her third year at the Naval Academy. I'd rather be here and ensure safe sailing for her generation, rather than running a boring private practice and wearing ties."

The Crisis Center team walked into the maze of ventilators, plastic tubing and folding cots in the center of the conference floor. Hundreds of family members sat in folding chairs and on supply boxes, anxiously awaiting any signs of improvement in their loved ones. There was a surprising quiet, considering the number of people, each with their own stories, crammed into close proximity under stressful conditions.

Doctors Mateo and Marshall supervised the administration of the last of the botulinum antitoxin to the patients on ventilatory assistance.

"We'll see if two doses are enough," Marshall thought aloud. "If they don't get better, we'll just have give them more as soon as we can get it."

"How do they determine what's in a vial, anyway?" asked Mateo.

"It's based on science, just not human science," admitted Marshall. "The amount to reverse botulism symptoms in rats is determined and then extrapolated to the weight of a human. The trivalent antitoxin actually has antibodies to A, B, and E toxins, but only the A is likely to cause a respiratory collapse. Since your testing indicates we're dealing with pure A toxin alone, we might need more of the antitoxin to neutralize it all."

"Look at that!" Mateo suddenly exclaimed to Marshall.

The physicians stood by the bedside of a twelve-year-old girl, who at twelve hours into antitoxin therapy was beginning to breathe on her own. Her long, dark hair moved slightly on her folding cot as her neck muscles were able to move her head for the first time in more than twenty-four hours. The fingers on her right hand began to move, and she was able to shift her eyes to the right to see the men who were saving her life.

"Thank you, Jesus," sighed Mateo as he breathed each shallow breath along with the young girl who gave them hope for miracles.

During the next hour, eight more people exhibited weak but life-sustaining breathing. Although their tired muscles tried to re-position arms and legs, only a flicker of movement occurred. An occasional toxin-affected patient coughed into his endotracheal tube as his diaphragm and chest muscles began to recover.

"We'll watch them for an hour," suggested Marshall, "and if they keep breathing, we'll pull the endotracheal tubes. As we remove the vents, we can hustle the vents over to the patients whose families are still squeezing Ambu bags."

Chapter 21

REPORT

Tehran; 13 September 2008

The door slid open to reveal the main laboratory workspace and the near-panicked face of his assistant, Jalil.

"Ah ... Doctor ... we have a visit from the General!" Jalil said with false enthusiasm.

General Madmudiyeh moved from his position to the right of the door and into Atoomb's view. His eyes traveled down the relaxed, Western clothing the scientist wore and then to the untied tennis shoes. The general scowled but said nothing.

"General," stammered Atoomb. "Thank you for your time. I trust you are pleased with the initial reports from Philadelphia?"

"The results are ... adequate," he said finally. "I pray that you are correct about the infectious phase that you have predicted."

His face showed little emotion but still carried a threat.

"Just give the agent three days, General," pleaded Atoomb.

"The counselors expect a complete and detailed record of the production of the germ," warned Madmudiyeh. "I will review the report at the end of this week."

Atoomb nodded glumly and planned yet another interruption in the work that he needed to accomplish.

A *detailed record*, thought the scientist, *makes me expendable.*

~

Yet Atoomb entered his report into the secure database of the factory's aged computer system.

"For four years," he wrote, "I worked in the Iranian biological weapons research program in the Hamadan laboratory. My supervisors in the lab were drawn from the Soviet scientists who came to Iran from the Russian *Biopreparat* bioweapons program.

"More than three thousand of these knowledgeable men and women had been left unemployed and starving by the economic collapse of the 'motherland' in 1991. The eighty-four scientists who entered Iran from Russia brought us information on plague, tularemia, anthrax, and smallpox, plus the critical techniques of keeping the biowarfare bacteria afloat in the air, where a human target can most easily inhale them. These scientists were experts in successful methods of distributing the germs by simple aerosol sprays from hidden containers or from fog generators placed in drone aircraft. They avoided the early mistakes of the Iraqis and refused to use explosive distributions, because the lethal element of surprise was lost.

"However, we were able to teach even these distinguished scientists," continued Atoomb, "about the processes of gene splicing and the introduction of new genetic traits into old germs. Our Hamadan laboratory results were only limited by the money available for equipment and enzyme reagents.

"On an April morning two years ago, two young representatives of the Islamic Republic's Committee of Counselors visited me in the Hamadan lab. These messengers were dressed in Western clothing but wore the keffiyeh."

Atoomb remembered how these powerful men were vastly different from the poor, white-coated scientists before them.

"'You have been selected to lead a great mission,' the representatives informed me. 'The details of the project you do not now need to know. You must prepare to depart for Tehran tomorrow morning with three of your most trusted workers. Your success will bring upon you the praise of Allah!'"

Atoomb's thoughts trailed off as he avoiding writing the rest of the representatives' words: "Your failure, the punishment of the counselors for all of your team."

"Two and a half years ago," Atoomb continued, "the Fathu al-Shamal facility underwent conversion to a biologic research laboratory, with an inner safety zone for the protection of our Islamic peoples. In decisions made through experience with the Soviets, we rejected the development and deployment of plague and anthrax germs, due to their slow incubation periods and the capacity for modern antibiotics to halt the infection. We had experience with viral agents such as smallpox, Ebola, and Marburg, but they were not yet stable weapons or reliable enough for use.

"Early in my training, I saw that toxins, produced in advance by pathogenic bacteria and ready to do Allah's work, would be the best pathway to strike the unbelievers. The production of a master toxin from a carefully constructed 'Jihad Germ' is the reason for the spending of such a large amount of our blessed funds.

"We began with samples of *Clostridium botulinum* germs ordered legally from the American Type Culture Collection by our Brothers in America through a U.S. company called the Biolimit Corporation. The company, according to its American paperwork, is a vaccine research and production factory. Its location in Pine Bluff, Arkansas, also the home of the U.S. Army's biologic study arsenal, causes many to think that our company is of the U.S. military. If the Americans visit the site listed as the home of Biolimit, they will only find an abandoned house and none of our Brothers."

Atoomb walked across the laboratory to gaze at the security of the sliding glass containment zone doors, behind which his scientific secrets rested. Full disclosure now could result in properly trained scientists duplicating his work … even if he were no longer around. He decided that he would provide enough detail to be convincing, but leave out enough detail to make the process impossible to reproduce.

"After we obtained and grew the Clostridium germs, we began to work on some of the problems with the toxin's production. The Clostridium germs are anaerobic, and exposure to the oxygen in open air kills them. We could never distribute the natural germ in the target country without loss of most of the cultures."

"Deoxyribonucleic acid, DNA, is the tool Allah has chosen to carry the gene information for life. Long, ribbon-like pairs of these nucleic acids line up to tell a living thing what it is to become. A simple virus has seven thousand pairs of these acids, while humans require more than three billion pairs to store the blueprints. Allah has given us the capacity to change these blueprints—and thus change the properties that living things exhibit.

"By using modern bioengineering, we were able to digest the Clostridium cultures with a gene cutter called a restriction endonuclease and obtain the DNA fragments which control the production of the botulism toxins. Although seven toxins occur naturally, only botulinum toxin A has the characteristics that Allah's work requires. The A toxin DNA was isolated by electroporesis and harvested.

"To produce our Jihad Germ, we selected a carrier bacterium that can live in air and is common in the human gastrointestinal tract, plus possesses natural immunity to many common antibiotics. We selected, through the Biolimit reference lab sources, a germ called Enterobacter and grew the germ in two of our new one-hundred-liter fermenters. This germ is naturally resistant to antibiotics that includes the drugs penicillin, erythromycin, and sulfa, plus cephalosporin and quinolone antibiotics. There are no known antibiotics taken by mouth that will kill the Enterobacter germ, and only a few antibiotics exist that will kill it when they are given intravenously."

Atoomb beamed with pride as he realized that the most critical aspect of the creation process would be virtually impossible without him.

"We then used techniques to make the Enterobacter germ cells more susceptible to incorporating new DNA, and our Micropulse 'gene gun' to fire the toxin DNA into the receiving cell. By then using an enzyme 'glue' called DNA ligase, we were able to paste the new DNA into the host germ cell. We then watched each of the new cultures until the Enterobacter germs began production of the toxin.

"After more than sixty failed culture attempts, we developed the masterpiece germ, which held wonderful antibiotic drug resistance, resistance to chlorination, and production of large amounts of Clostridium botulinum toxin A. We now have over three thousand liters of the descendants of this germ and have successful animal tests demonstrating their ability to do Allah's will.

"The Enterobacter germ is a natural contaminant of water supplies," Atoomb went on, "as evidenced by the death of over four thousand soldiers at the Andersonville prison during the American Civil War. These deaths came from naturally occurring Enterobacter dysentery, not our Enterobacter super germ carrying the genes to also produce large amounts of botulinum toxin. The world has never seen the power of the infectious agent that now rests in the hands of Allah."

Chapter 22

THE BUREAU

Philadelphia; 13 September 2008

"No update me," prodded Special Agent in Charge Wells as he stirred his coffee on the afternoon of September 13th. Wells, forty-eight, overweight, and nearing the end of a career as an FBI special agent, was in a supremely bad mood. He had not only been awake for more than forty hours, but the entire federal investigation system expected his initial findings *today*. He sat with Agents Deason and Landrum at a table in the FBI's Philadelphia field office, in the Green Building on Arch Street. An adjacent conference room bustled with the agents, computers, and the constantly ringing phones of an investigative agency in high gear.

"Well, sir," reported Deason after a pause for dramatic effect, "We are actively investigating in several directions and tracking items of interest. Deason, not likely to forget Krause's

stinging rebuke while in the command trailer, wanted perpetrators; and wanted them without allowing the incident
command structure in on the publicity.

"We began by looking at possible responsible organizations," Deason reported, "including Aryan, Islamic, and Klan.
Our covert contacts in the Aryan Brotherhood have no information on the attack, and the Ku Klux Klan is pissed about the
attack, since they are 'loyal Americans.' The materials from
the New York truck were turned over to the lab at Quantico,
and we anticipate information about the tank's content in
two to three days.

"In the Islamic arena, we located five area mosques, but
one stands out like a sore thumb. In reviewing the 990's for
tax-exempt organizations, we found the numbers interesting.
Four of the five mosques in the metro area reported a tax-
free income of between $75,000 and $200,000 a year, yet the
fifth, the Al-Douri Mosque, received a whopping $3.8 million
in donations from its 220 members. The mosque also has an
associated charitable group named the Delaware Bay Benevolence Fund, also based here in Philadelphia."

He went on.

"The NSA intercepted an encrypted cell phone call in
Arabic yesterday morning; with content noting that 'the early
reports are favorable' as the speaker addressed an unknown
contact traveling in Tennessee. The cell phone that originated
the call is registered to the Delaware Bay Benevolence Fund.
We have created a list of four persons of interest who seem to
have leadership positions. We are now tracking down these
individuals for questioning here at the operations center."

Agent Landrum continued the brief for the Agent in
Charge. "We performed a detailed crime scene investigation
at Pumping Station A, with attention to latent prints and the
tire-tread features of the truck. We obtained two partial foot-
prints in blood, but no suspect fingerprints, only glove marks
and smears. Several latent human hairs were recovered and

have been sent to the lab, along with samples of hair from the four decedents."

Landrum continued.

"Measurements of the truck's tread width and wheelbase yielded information that is helpful. The tread pattern was consistent with the most common truck tire size, an 11R 22.5; however, the wheelbase was relatively short, at 160 inches. There were also oil spots from two different locations beneath the truck. The Hoover Center experts tell us that the truck's wheelbase, which is shorter than a Mack or Kenworth, is most likely an older International."

"Okay," pressed Wells. "How many older Internationals are registered in metro Philadelphia?"

"There are thirty-eight Internationals more than five years old registered within a hundred-mile radius, and we have agents tracking them all to see how many are still in use," Landrum informed him.

"We are also looking at possible sources of botulinum germs," resumed Deason, "and have found that the only common commercial source of the germ in the United States is a nonprofit organization in Virginia called the American Type Culture Collection. Our preliminary contact indicates that more than four thousand university and pharmaceutical labs ordered the germ over the last five years."

"Four thousand!" exclaimed Wells. "Why the hell do that many people need a toxic germ?"

Landrum shrugged. "It seems that low doses of the toxin are being used by doctors to relax wrinkles, and there's money in looking young."

"I need results—the Terrorist Threat Center is already breathing down my neck," Wells frowned. "Get a court order for a 'freeze and seize' on this mosque's financial records, computers, and paper files. I want someone to physically inspect each of the old Internationals on the list and interview the owners. I want an update tomorrow on the footprint and hair evidence."

"Got it, Chief," said Deason as he updated the schedule on his PDA.

As the agents departed the Agent in Charge update, Landrum stopped near the door.

"Sir?" Landrum asked Wells. "How much of this investigation will be released to the Philadelphia incident command structure?"

"None of it," answered Wells curtly. "We can't afford to have the fire department and a bunch of hospital administrators scaring our rabbits into their holes."

∿

By ten a.m. on September 13, FBI Special Agents Morris and Clinton, along with a Chem-Bio Incident Response Force lance corporal had looked at more old trucks than they thought possible in a little over nine hours.

"Hey, Morrie," puzzled Clinton, "we got only twelve trucks left; you think the thing was even registered in Philadelphia?"

"Hell, I don't know," replied Morris. "Only a few of them are even still running, and I sure haven't seen anything suspicious."

The fruitless search had mostly turned up wrecking-yard trucks and a few trucks that were still running, and owned by old men with small businesses. Nevertheless, the Marine corporal had assisted the special agents in using SMART membranes to screen the each of the trucks for toxin residue—and drew a blank on each.

"Well, maybe we'll find the rest before midnight," hoped Clinton, who was clearly unimpressed with his assignment in the investigation.

∿

The morning of September 14 brought surprise for Imam Derwish of the Al-Douri Mosque. Ten minutes after he unlocked the door, made his morning tea and began to open the mail, four agents wearing body armor labeled "FBI" and carrying assault weapons joined him.

"You cannot be here," Derwish spat. "This is a holy place!"

"This 'holy place' is within the United States of America and is subject to its laws," Deason responded coolly. "You have the opportunity to voluntarily accompany us for discussion about the operation of this mosque," he added, "or depart in handcuffs, under arrest."

"On what charge?" fumed Derwish.

"We'll begin with support of international terrorism, money laundering, and accessory to murder," Deason smiled, "and go from there."

Silently, Imam Derwish rose and accompanied the armed men to their waiting, unmarked Ford. As the five men walked through the still-darkened mosque, the imam saw more than a dozen impeccably suited FBI agents load the three office computers and all of the file drawers into the rear of waiting vans. The raid was over in less than an hour, with four agents left behind to transport any late arriving mosque members to their equally voluntary discussions."

~

Special Agent Landrum scanned the four-thousand-item list of recipients of *Clostridium botulinum* germs, which had been provided by the American Type Culture Collection. He placed recognized universities and major drug companies to the rear of his suspect list and concentrated on the smaller labs and companies whose names carried no public recognition. The culling process still left him with more than twelve hundred entities to investigate.

Landrum called two agents, who held the least seniority,

with a smile.

"I have a little job for you,: Landrum began. "I want you to contact these highlighted companies and notify them of an ongoing investigation into the criminal use of botulism germs. The information they are to provide includes dates and amounts of Clostridium that they purchased, and the names of individuals in their organization responsible for any Clostridium research. We need the names, phone numbers, and e-mail addresses of the all of the scientists who have had access to the toxin-producing germs. Give each company twelve hours to comply."

"And if they don't?" asked Adams.

"Then you'll be making a few visits," Landrum grinned. "You'll also make a visit if the dates and amounts are not in agreement with this sales printout or if the company seems to have forgotten details of its research in the botulism area. I'll need an update in twenty-four hours and will get you additional manpower for the road trips."

"Will do," responded one of the junior agents. The pair retreated into the bustle of the adjacent operations center, one shaking his head and the other mumbling quiet curses.

～

SAC Wells completed the encrypted e-mail report to the FBI's counterterrorism division and pushed the "Send" button.

"I don't know if this new terrorism fighting system will help or hinder," he admitted to Landrum.

After his information underwent review by the Counter Terrorism Division, it would be directed to the Terrorist Threat Integrative Center. The theory of centrally locating information about terrorists was sound, but who knew about the practical application of information flow across three different government agencies. The Threat Integrative Center included members from the FBI's Counterterrorism Division, the CIA's Counterterrorism Center, and the Department of Homeland Security's Information Analysis and Infrastructure Protection Directorate. The information sharing across federal agencies had proven problematic during 9/11, and the reality within the new organization might just be another layer of bureaucracy in which to lose valuable information.

"Hell, I ought to know," Wells grumbled, as he remembered the Bureau's six-month-long misplacement of his retirement account funds.

Chapter 23

AMELIORATION

Philadelphia; 13 September 2008

Outside of Jefferson University Hospital's ER entrance, a Marine staff sergeant serving as the non-commissioned offer in charge of decontamination procedures sat on the patient rollers that ran through the midline of the Crisis Center decontamination tent.

"So what you want me to do now?" the decontamination private assigned asked.

"You can come off your self-contained breathing gear, open your hood and stand by," instructed the sergeant. "Have Private Williams post by the entrance in full 'B' suit, and he can tell us to suit up if we get more patients."

With no new casualties over the last several hours, removing their hoods would save the sixty-minute pressurized air tanks, which would mean less to refill later. The new lightweight plastic suits were warm, but they beat the heavy butyl rubber suits the team had started with three years earlier. The olive-green suit was lightweight Tyvek and had built-in gloves and boots. The suits made the team look like Michelin men, with their oversized plastic hoods and the bulky air tank enclosed in the back of the suit adding to the strangeness of their appearance. While enclosed in the outfit, the Marines felt the slight pressure of compressed air that not only enabled them to breathe, but also forced away any germs trying to enter the suit. The sergeant had stopped smoking; it was just too much trouble to light up with the majority of his time spent in the suit.

If patient decontaminations were finished at the hospital, he would break some of his guys out of the potentially contaminated red zone and send them to the tourist areas in the Historic District to ensure that they had been sprayed and rinsed. Maybe they would get the chance to go back to the Old City as customers before leaving on the return trip to Indian Head.

~

Dr. Ron Raines had never assumed a shift with only two patients on the board. He took over the care of a nursing home patient admitted for pneumonia and a child who had fallen from a grocery store shopping buggy. It was difficult to believe that a mere twenty-four hours ago, he was adrift in a sea of critically ill toxin victims, and tonight, there were none. Major Tower had brought word of twelve patients who were now off ventilatory support after receiving the botulinum antitoxin therapy given in the Crisis Center. Maybe there really were answers to prayers.

"I've never seen it so—" Raines began, but the crystalline-blue, laughing eyes of Karen Winslow interrupted him.

"Never, ever, say the Q word in an ER!" she chastised with a grin. "It will only bring you bad luck."

Raines took the advice with a good-natured smile and sat down at the triage nursing desk to answer his backlog of e-mail.

"So what's up with you and your Prince Charming?" Karen asked as Christie stocked intravenous fluids into the hall warmer.

"The prince turned out to be a toad," Christie admitted. "It seems he needed cocaine for his 'professional edge' and that he was in hock for the Jag and the Rolex. I'm thinking of taking up a life of celibacy."

Raines deleted junk e-mail from airlines, pet medicine companies, and the reunion services that promised to find all of his dear old friends in Arkansas. He was left with only four e-mails from real people and a new awareness of the ratio of wheat to chaf in a modern world of information.

His first real email was from a young man in Monterrey, Mexico; a young man that Raines had never met. Raines knew a former Ranger, now called Father Rodriquez, and budgeted three hundred dollars a month to send to the priest to support the education of four young boys. Father Rodriguez provided refuge from the streets and a future that otherwise, would not have existed. The young man used the priest's "computadora" to thank Raines, and assure that he would study hard and become a doctor someday. Raines smiled, and was able to forget briefly the evil that lurked in the shadows of his new home city. He thought he had a special affinity for the street kids—after all, he was just a street kid, too.

Chapter 24

HOUSTON

Texas; 14 September 2008

On Friday evening, the two Faithful performed the ritual ablution, followed by the *Salaat* with the group of forty Muslim worshippers. Ahmed Madawi was the Faithful's spokesman and mounted the speaker's platform, where he stood nervously before the microphone.

"My Brothers and I are grateful for your hospitality to travelers so far from Mecca. We are students and Faithful followers of the Qur'an and speak to you this evening with humble hearts.

"In 1924, when Ataturk established a secular government in Turkey, our Muslim Brotherhood of al-Kharij was born. The Brotherhood fought against those who would turn their backs on the true glory of Islam. During this period, Sayyid Qutb, an Egyptian who braved life in the lands of the infidel, left us the *Ma'alim fi el-Tareek*, the book of *Signs Along the Road*, to learn from. He gave his life for its publication.

"He lets us know important truths, and I would like to share with you his words."

Ahmed began reading aloud from the text.

"'Today we are living like heathens, just like the days before Islam, in the way people act, the world's culture, and what they believe and think. It is all heathenism. Even in the Islamic world, the people's thinking and their laws are all far from the true Islam. The way that life is lived today is an insult to Allah and his authority on earth. This idolatrous world gives the authority of Allah to humans as if they were God. These heathens are not like the ones before Islam, but far worse.'"

Ahmed continued reading.

"Today's heathens reverence and honor man-made constitutions, laws, and principles. They disregard Allah's law and His constitution for life. We should immediately eliminate this pagan influence and the heathen pressure on our world. We must overturn this current society, with its culture and leadership of infidels. This is our first priority: to shake and change the foundations of heathens. We must destroy whatever conflicts with true Islam. We should get out from under the bondage of what keeps us from living in the ways that Allah wants us to live.'"

Ahmed closed the book and paused.

"Although this was written in Egypt more than fifty years ago, it has never been so true as now, when the infidel governments of America, Europe, and Israel lead people away from Allah. My Brothers and I believe in the tools of Jihad to change our Islamic people. We will join in the coming Jihad using the tools and planning that Allah asks of us. Allah Akbar."

Imam Hafiz stood with a tall, dark-complexioned man at the rear of the room. The stranger wore an American three-piece suit of tan fabric, and his glasses shielded his eyes from any observer. The unnamed man's face wore the mask of too many battles, and there was an air of pride in his movements.

As Madawi neared the back of the room, Mohammed and Farouk joined him, and when together, the imam motioned them closer. Beside the imam stood a granite faced, muscular man wearing a tan suit, and despite being indoors, wore dark glasses.

"My Faithful Brothers," the imam spoke to the three young men, "there are many ways in which you can be of service to Allah. Tonight we have a great soldier of the Sword of Islam visiting, and I ask you to speak further with him."

The unsmiling stranger led the three Faithful to their dormitory room and closed the door behind them.

"For now," began the stranger, "I will be known to you as Mahesh. You speak the truth of our upcoming battles for Islam, and I have an opportunity for two of you to consider. I am truly sorry, but our brother Mohammed, who has only one eye, is not to be accepted for training.

"In Arizona, we have developed a training camp whose goal is to teach much of the tools of warfare that you describe. The training continues for six months and gives the mujahideen warrior a deeper knowledge of weapons and explosives, assassination, hostage operations, and communication networks.

"The center is called Al-Aqsa," continued Mahesh. "If you desire to be trained, you will be paid as the dedicated workers that you are, and you will make many professional contacts that may become useful in your future. Only a few are selected, but I feel you may be of great service to Allah in the al-Aqsa Martyr's Brigade."

Chapter 25

THE DRYER

Tehran; 14 September 2008

Dr. Khalid Atoomb smiled at the possibilities as he performed the final inspection of the installation of the laboratory's new AeroPure (rotary) vacuum dryer.

Surely these results will make the old goat happy! he thought as he peered through the high-impact face shield of his containment suit. The unit had room temperature drying capacity and triple-pass drying phases, and it filtered air intake to ensure the purity of the product. Atoomb was certain the bacterial agent would have much higher survivability in this unit than if he had chosen freeze-drying or thermal-drying equipment.

He walked to the photoelectric eye at the Zone Three lab's exit and moved through the doorway into Zone Two.

Atoomb slid off the containment suit and dropped it into

the decontamination chute, then stripped off his gloves and discarded them. He stepped quickly into the shower as his mind circled around the new potential of the equipment.

The American mail, he thought as he toweled himself dry and then dropped the towel into the decontamination chute.

Atoomb pulled on blue jeans and a T-shirt and covered the ensemble with a worn lab coat. He slipped on his sneakers and planned to tie them after leaving Zone Two.

Atoomb entered the laboratory workroom to find General Madmudiyeh waiting. The old warrior again noticed Atoomb's untied shoes and then looked directly into the scientist's eyes. He paused and looked at the AeroPure manual that lay open upon the laboratory table.

"And this expensive new toy," he said as his eyes narrowed. "Tell me again why you spent a million rials for it."

"The vacuum dryer," Atoomb began yet again, "will enable the weapon to reach an entirely new level of dispersion and effectiveness. By carefully drying the live cultures, we can produce a fine powder or tablets that contain the Jihad Germ in incredible concentrations. The simple addition of water will restore the organism back to its fully infectious nature."

"And this is worth a million rials?" growled General Madmudiyeh.

"General, think of the possibilities," Atoomb pleaded desperately. "A dry powder of highly concentrated germ culture could be compressed into tablets and dropped by the handful into a city's reservoir, where it would be released over months. A dry powder is a form that an operative could sprinkle over an infidel salad bar. A dry powder could be sent through the American mail system."

"We will see, Atoomb," said the General flatly. "You have spent a very great sum of money for your playthings."

"The money will allow us a great victory …"

Atoomb trailed off as the general turned on his heel and stalked from the room. The scientist wiped the sweat from his brow with the sleeve of his lab coat. He sank into a chair and looked at Jalil.

"We start the drying experiments this afternoon," Atoomb said, but his thoughts continued: *and I pray that the techniques are successful.*

That was the problem with working in a hidden laboratory, deep within in a program whose hallmark was secrecy. He would never be able to discuss his work with other scientists, to learn from their experience and share his knowledge. If he produced the greatest advances known to the history of science, he would still lie in an unmarked grave—and after living the life of a pauper.

Chapter 26

TRAILS

Philadelphia; 14 September 2008

The Al-Douri's Imam Derwish appeared genuinely confused at becoming a "person of interest" to the FBI. He sat stiffly before the video camera in the Green Building's FBI conference room as Special Agent Landrum questioned him.

"Tell us about the funding of your mosque and how your money is spent," Landrum demanded.

"We are funded by many sources," replied the dazed Imam, "and the funds, of course, go for the mosque and its upkeep, plus religious education in this and our outreach areas, in addition to numerous charitable causes."

"Tell me about your 'many funding sources,'" continued Landrum.

"We are funded through the contributions of our Faithful

members," answered Derwish, "and we hold a yearly conference that raises funds. We receive funds from various Islamic
support groups and several philanthropic and governmental
organizations."

"Which Islamic support groups?" Landrum pressed.

"We are supported by the International Institute of Islamic
Thought, the Muslim Brotherhood, the International Benevolence Fund, and the Global Relief Foundation," the imam
recited. "We have felt Allah's goodness in fundraising during
the last three years."

"Who is the MLF?" continued Landrum.

"The Muslim Liberation Front," Derwish said.

"Why would a Palestinian organization be interested in a
mosque in faraway America?"

"Muslims are kind and caring people who only desire the
spread of the word of Allah," came the imam's humble answer.
"We receive funds from Harvard University's Hauser Center,
the National Crime Prevention Council's Outreach to New
Americans, from the U.S. Labor Department's Aid to Needy
Families, and we have a community service block grant from
the State of Pennsylvania."

Landrum was amazed.

"These governmental sources of funds, such as the Labor
Department and the state, are in addition to the federal benefits of being a tax-exempt organization?" he asked. "Are these
funds included in your tax-exempt financial reports?"

"Yes, of course," responded Derwish.

"How much money have you been provided by organizations outside of the United States?" Landrum asked.

"I have no firm figures without an exhaustive search of our
donations for the year," answered the imam.

"And where does all this money go, Imam Derwish?"

"We support our mosque and its employees, Islamic educational programs in Pennsylvania and New Jersey, a published
newsletter, and several Islamic charitable activities."

"What charitable activities do you support?" asked Landrum.

"We clothe the needy, feed the poor, and house some of the new members of our religious faith," Derwish responded.

"And this costs more than three million dollars a year?" exploded Landrum.

There was no response from the now uncomfortable religious leader.

"What is the Delaware Bay Benevolence Fund?" Landrum asked pointedly.

"The fund is a charitable group who provides for needy Muslims throughout Pennsylvania, New Jersey, and New York," the imam told him. "It is headed by Dr. Ali Zarif, a prominent local educator affiliated with Philadelphia Community College."

"And who controls how the funds are distributed?" Landrum pressed.

"That is the responsibility of Dr. Zarif, who is now caring for hundreds new to the Islamic faith," Derwish proudly concluded. "He is aided by a benevolence committee of three leaders who share the decisions for the expenditures."

～

Dr. Ali Zarif sat uncomfortably at the end of a field office conference table, flanked by Agents Landrum and Deason, with Wells, the Special Agent in Charge, remaining in the background. Zarif fidgeted under the scrutiny of a running videotape. He had been given only the option of a voluntary discussion or arrest, and he had chosen the former.

"Dr. Zarif," droned Landrum, "tell us of your activities on behalf of the Al-Douri Mosque."

"I am merely a teacher for my computer science students and a Faithful follower of my God and his mosque," came the humble reply from the bespectacled professor.

"Since it is illegal to support religious activities with governmental funds, how are federal and state funds being used for the support of the activities of your mosque?" Landrum continued.

"I am aware of funds for needy families and wellness grants," replied Zarif. "However, these funds are carefully allocated to the betterment of the poor and do not support our religious activities."

"And how do you better the poor without furthering the mosque's religious agenda?" asked Landrum with visible irritation.

"We keep no secrets regarding the fact that the funds for food and housing are from the mosque's sphere of influence and that we wish our Brothers to find God. However, the governmental funds are placed directly into the Delaware Bay Benevolence Fund and never used for the support of the mosque, for its newsletter, or for the payment of its staff," Zarif defended.

"What is your knowledge of the MLF?" demanded Landrum.

"I've never heard of that organization," Zarif replied.

"Then how did you know that the letters stood for an organization?" quizzed Landrum.

There was no reply.

"Tell us about your activities on behalf of the Delaware Bay Benevolence Fund," Landrum pounded, with his anger at the taxpayer funding of possible illegal activities poorly disguised.

"I am chairman of the fund," Zarif responded. "and direct this charitable vehicle for the support of needy Muslims who live in the Eastern United States."

"What projects do you fund?"

"The mosque pays for the Islamic educational funds in Pennsylvania and New Jersey," noted Zarif, "and a newsletter for the mosque Faithful. The religious education is funded by the charity of Muslims in many lands. As we already discussed,

federal and state funds are channeled through the Benevolence Fund only to feed the poor and house the homeless."

"What is the total amount of charity funded by the Delaware Bay Benevolence Fund over the last year?"

"Around two million," Zarif reported quietly.

"That's a lot of charity, Doctor," Landrum said bluntly.
"Tell me about the Benevolence Fund's $11,000 payment to
Landers Trucking of Phoenix, Arizona."

Zarif's eyes widened in surprise.

How did these infidel fools discover the truck purchase so quickly?
he wondered.

"Ah … the Benevolence Fund purchased a truck and trailer
to distribute clothing and food to needy families, but the costs
to repair it for use were prohibitive," explained Zarif. "Thus,
the vehicle is being sold at auction," he added in a voice with
a noticeable tremor.

"What kind of truck?" prodded Landrum.

"A 1994 International," Zarif replied truthfully.

"Where and when was the vehicle sold?"

"Faithful members are arranging the sale, and I'm not
aware of the location of the truck, or if it has already been
sold."

"Which members are responsible for the sale?"

"Moustafa Saleeb," Zarif said, providing the first false name
that came to his mind.

Landrum zeroed in for the attack.

"Do you fund terrorist activities inside of the United
States?" he asked.

"Of course not," answered Zarif haughtily. "I am an American citizen."

"Do you fund terrorist activities outside of the United
States?" continued Landrum.

"No," defended Zarif, and then with consideration, added
enough detail to avoid contradicting the things that the FBI
might already know. "Some of the funds raised in our mosque

symposia are given to Muslim charitable organizations in other areas of the world, but I have no specific knowledge of how these funds are used. However, the American Muslim community is not a supporter of terrorist activities."

"How long have you been in the United States?" asked Landrum threateningly, despite his knowledge of the answer.

"For twelve years," answered Zarif. "I came to the United States on a student visa in 1995 and became a citizen four years ago."

"I have no further questions for you today, Doctor," Landrum said. "However, you are to remain within the state and available for additional questioning. Your departure from the state would be cause for immediate arrest."

Zarif rose shakily and exited the conference room without a glance or word for the agents.

"You know that's our man," muttered Agent in Charge Wells quietly—and unnecessarily.

"All we can pin on him now is receiving a lot of money for the Benevolence Fund and purchasing a truck suspected in a major crime," Landrum admitted with a frustrated shrug. "We've bugged his lines and just placed a Stealth GPS device under his car, out of sight above the gas tank. We'll grab his computers tonight when he's not expecting us."

"Do you think he'll run?" asked Deason.

"Of course he'll run," Landrum answered. "And we'll let our rabbit take us to his lair."

Chapter 27

FLIGHT

Pennsylvania to Maryland; 14-15 September 2008

Dr. Ali Zarif pushed the "Enter" key and confirmed the inquiry of his overly helpful software. Yes, he was quite sure he really wanted to format the hard drive and destroy its data.

"All data on C: drive will be destroyed," was the program's final warning before it began to churn through the hard drive and leave the computer's memory a blank.

Zarif's mind raced as he planned the sanitization of the small, south Philadelphia rental house. His address book contained the only written backup copies of the hundreds of names and e-mail addresses through which he kept in touch with the Brotherhood of Islamic Jihad. He had safely packed it in the duffel bag, along with his prayer rug and the AK-74. He left off the silencer, since mobility was now more important than silence. He slipped the Makarov pistol into his waistband and began to pour gasoline onto the bedroom floor. Zarif dropped a lighted match and watched as the purifying flame began to grow on the piled clothing and crawl across the carpeted floor. He slipped from the house as the clothing trail reached the gasoline-soaked carpet and burst into flames that licked the bedroom walls.

Ali Zarif stopped in the garage long enough to drop a second match into the fuel beneath the Loring Valve van and hurried into the night long before the flames reached the plastic containers of gasoline in the cargo space and seats of the vehicle. He walked rapidly to the burgundy Buick parked at the end of the driveway and drove away without looking back.

Special Agent Morris picked up the VHS transceiver and spoke in clipped but directing phrases.

"He's on the move, and I need the Philadelphia fire department ASAP for evidence protection."

"On the way," came the terse reply.

~

Zarif entered Interstate 95 South, leaving Philadelphia forever in the past.

They are uncovering too much for me to stay, he reasoned, and began to think of financial mechanisms to launder and recover the copious cash sitting in the Benevolence account.

They knew of the truck and at least some of the sources of the Benevolence account funding, and it was only a matter of time until they tracked the rental of the Arsenault plant and the deeper hidden ties to Biolimit. Spending a few weeks lost in Houston seemed the most logical measure until he could exit the country. As he drove, he opened the duffel and placed the assault rifle on the seat beside him.

As he attempted to follow the minds of the investigators, suddenly his eyes grew wide.

"What if they are tracking the vehicle!" he exclaimed.

At just after one a.m., he looked for the next exit, sped off the interstate and entered the parking lot of an all-night Chevron station. He filled the vehicle's tank and paid at the pump. Next, he pulled the Buick onto the "air and water" area of the parking lot and left the vehicle running. He retrieved a knife from beneath the seat and pried the rearview mirror from the inside of the windshield. As he circled the vehicle, he picked up the station's air compressor hose and began the ruse of examining the vehicle tires.

Where are you? he thought, enjoying this investigative game of chess. He used the mirror to peer beneath the fender wells and under the chassis of the car.

With only one e-mail to Imam Hafiz and the computer destroyed, the FBI will find the suburbs of Houston as obscure as the Amazon, he smiled as he searched for the GPS unit.

Texas is a big state ...

At the left rear of the vehicle, mounted on the chassis above the gas tank, he saw the four-inch rectangular tracking unit with its rubberized antenna.

"Aha, there you are!" he said as he plucked the magnetic unit from its hiding place. Zarif walked toward the station but dropped his keys beside a parked Toyota truck. As he bent to retrieve the keys, he slapped the GPS unit beneath on the chassis below the driver's door. Some unbeliever on his way home from work would lead the FBI on a nice, long and merry chase. After purchasing gasoline and a soft drink, he reentered the Buick, laughed to himself, and headed northwest on Interstate 476. Leaving Philadelphia in his past, the signs pointed him toward Allentown, Wilkes-Barre and northern Pennsylvania, the last direction that someone headed south might choose.

～

The fire lieutenant walked into the still smoldering South Philly house. The garage was a total loss, but the Loring Valve logo had still been visible on the burned shell of the van.

"I'm not sure why all the federal interest," he remarked to the driver of Philadelphia Engine12, "but looks like they got what they wanted."

The firefighters watched as six agents exited the house with a smoke-singed computer system, wrapped glassware, and even a shrink-wrapped coffee table.

"Betcha it's got something to do with the poison attack," remarked the fire department driver.

〜

"He bought twenty-one dollars in gas at a Chevron and is headed north on I-95," relayed Deason as he watched the GPS blip on the computer screen.

"I don't believe it," Landrum said. "The NSA intercept shows his boys were headed south and in Tennessee at the time of the call. Launch the bird!"

At Philadelphia's Penn Landing Heliport, Special Agent Taylor pressed the earpiece deeper into his left ear and gave the pilot an overhead twirling motion with his right fingers. The dark blue FBI Bell 201B helicopter began its rotor spin-up as the agent and his spotter/sniper team climbed into the vibrating cockpit.

"This is an ID and break-off only, not a take-down," Taylor relayed to the man holding the M-107 sniper rifle. Coordination and planning was of great importance when dealing with a combination of man, weapon, and AN/PVS 10 sight that could launch a .50-caliber round accurately enough to reach out and touch someone more than a mile away.

The chopper lifted off, dipped its nose to the north, and rapidly moved toward the GPS coordinates flashing across the screen of Taylor's laptop. In less than ten minutes, they dropped to two hundred feet, over the surprised figure of a middle-aged man driving a rusting Toyota truck.

"The vehicle is a negative for the suspect," Taylor said into his encrypted cell phone. "It looks like the suspect switched the GPS unit to an old truck."

"Break off and head south on I-95," Landrum replied. "Burgundy 2001 Buick. Find him!"

"Roger," complied Taylor, and the helicopter banked through a 180-degree turn.

~

As the helicopter's rotors began to reverberate from the buildings of the Washington metro area, Taylor's spirits sagged with the knowledge that there was just too much area to cover.

"Dammit, we friggin lost him!" Taylor reported to Landrum in frustration.

"We already have the Pennsylvania State Police looking for him, and I'm calling the Maryland state boys and the D.C. city cops now. He will have to travel south on 95 or farther to the west on Interstate 81. We cannot let this man get away!"

Taylor looked carefully at the map and the major cities on I-95 and then directed his pilot to bank to the west to intercept Interstate 81.

The best route is 476 west to Interstate 81 from Philadelphia ... and then 81 rockets southeast, avoiding of all the major cities, thought Taylor hopefully. *That'd be the route I'd choose if I wanted to put mileage behind me!*

Ali Zarif drove seventy-eight miles-per-hour; the maximum speed that he felt would avoid the attention of any local police forces. He turned onto Interstate 76 West, skated across the Pennsylvania Turnpike, and crossed the Susquehanna River as the sun began to rise and burn away the fog that hovered over several small islands and the solemn gray block remnants of a Civil War era stone bridge. He turned south on Interstate 81, and he crossed the Maryland state line near Hagerstown just before eight a.m. He glanced at his Palm Pilot map and smiled at the long, uninterrupted ribbon of southeastern road in which one could drive for hundreds of miles without nearing a city. He checked the battery on the radar detector and found the green light reassuring.

Even if they are setting up roadblocks, the fools will leave their radar guns on, he reasoned. It was too easy to outsmart these lawmen; men who thought they had been placed in charge of the behavior of others.

Chapter 28

FLAME

Philadelphia; 14–15 September 2008

When Raines reported for an ER shift, the parking lot always told him what to expect. This evening as he pulled the Harley into Jefferson's parking lot, he knew that something was wrong again. There were five ambulances parked in the entrance bay, and a crowd of worried family members talked by the triage doors.

"Six new toxin cases, all over the last two hours," Matt Kindred greeted Raines breathlessly. "We've already called Dr. Marshall and the CBIRF team and requested a recheck on the water supply."

"Oh, hell ... not again," Raines said, a sentiment Kindred shared.

The green-tiled walls of Jefferson University Hospital's ER had seen too much—too many poor and homeless, too much pain and death. The electronics and medical equipment, the drugs and medical supplies were all the newest and the best. The faces of those in health care training were all new ... but the walls were old and experienced. Yet, no health care facility in the world had experienced the level of death and illness presented to this national bastion of care on September 11, 2008. Now, on the 14th, the nightmare was beginning again.

Raines walked into the resuscitation bay to see four intubated patients, three of whom were on the last ventilators still available at Jefferson. Rooms Two, Three, and Four contained patients with arm and facial weakness, requiring monitoring of oxygen saturation for signs of respiratory failure. The hall held frightened people with facial weakness only.

"It's going to be a long night," Raines said aloud to Karen at the triage desk.

"Someone must have said the Q word."

He put in a page for Dr. Case.

"Just wanted to warn you that the triage tent is about to be hit again," he said quietly.

Raines rapidly moved from patient to patient, documenting on the charts the times of his exams and the presence of weakened muscle groups. After he had seen and documented all patients, he would repeat the process to catch any further development of weakness.

"Something is different this time," he remarked to Christie. "Almost all of these patients had a slower onset and less severe symptoms. Also, they are reporting diarrhea and have fever. There is more dehydration than we saw in the initial attack. This is different from the toxin exposure; this looks like an active infection. Get blood cultures on everyone with a fever, and start Ringer's lactate on those with an elevated heart rate or low blood pressure. We have to assume the diarrhea is infectious, and even touching a patient might spread the germ."

Just after eight p.m., Major Tower walked through triage

to report his findings to Raines.

"The water is still okay, Ron," he puzzled. "Do you want to look for food sources?"

"Can't see how any food source could be this widespread," Raines answered. "This must be a flare of something left over from the initial attack. We need Marshall's involvement ASAP. I'll page him."

As Tower walked down the hall to leave, he noticed a frightened family in Room Twelve. A young mother and a son received intravenous fluids, while a young girl sat solemnly in the chair beneath an x-ray view box.

As Christie hurried down the emergency department hallway, she saw the look of concern on Tower's face and gave him the background on the family. The father died in the toxin attack, and now two of the three household survivors were sick.

"I'm not sure what we'll do with the daughter while her mother and brother are being treated," she said.

Tower saw the pale, dehydrated faces of the young mother and son and thought about his own family at home.

They're just good people going about their own lives, only to have someone's political agenda snatch away the things most important to them, he thought.

~

After two hours, Raines had twenty-four patients under his management, with only two more requiring intubation and Ambu bag assistance. Raines entered Room Fourteen to see a pretty nineteen-year-old blonde lying on the gurney and a distraught father standing at the bedside.

"Please, you've got to help her," the father pleaded. "We lost her mother just three days ago."

The young woman was experiencing facial muscle weakness, blurred vision, abdominal cramps and fever, and she reported, with some embarrassment, that she had experienced diarrhea since noon.

"I'm Mandy McConnell," said the obviously ill young lady, barely able to exhibit a brave smile.

Raines examined her carefully and found her oxygen saturation level and the palpation of her abdomen to be reassuring. He ordered intravenous fluids plus medications for cramps and nausea.

Christy departed to retrieve the medications while Dr. Raines reassured Mr. McConnell.

"We're going to throw everything in the book at this problem," he said. "We'll take care of her."

~

"Take a look at these," Raines said with knitted brows as he handed a stack of laboratory reports to Chris Richards, his ER coverage partner.

"They all have high white blood counts and mild acidosis," he remarked, "and that is new for this disease process."

Richards studied the reports and saw that, in fact, that all of the patients had white blood counts in excess of 14,000, and about half had elevations to more than 20,000 infection-fighting cells, almost double the normal levels in a healthy patient . Decreases in the serum bicarbonate levels revealed the presence of acidosis, likely from infection or significant dehydration.

"So what do you think is going on, other than more fluid loss than before?" asked Richards.

"Almost all of the new cases have diarrhea," Raines explained, "and the white counts make it look like an active bacterial infection may be the problem. You just can't account for all of it with botulinum toxin. I think the Clostridium germs are now growing in these patients."

"Then I don't understand why the signs of infection didn't show up on the first attack and why Clostridium bugs weren't seen on the Polymerase Chain Reaction studies," Richards said. "The bacteria have to be there somewhere."

Raines dialed the number for Marshall's digital pager, and was relieved that the infectious disease specialist called back within seconds.

"Doc, this now looks more like an active infectious disease," reported Raines. "We just can't figure out why we don't see the germ on the PCR studies. Do you want to change the antibiotic coverage?"

"Ciprofloxacin and ampicillin should cover Clostridium well," reassured Marshall. "How's your supply holding up?"

"We're running low on both, and we were already out of ventilators before this flare started," said Raines.

"If you run out of the antibiotics, I'd try gentamicin plus sulfa drugs," Marshall suggested. "I'll get in touch with Slidell and push him for antibiotics from local pharmacies. We can give the meds orally to those who are still walking and talking."

"We have forty thousand doses of the *Clostridium botulinum* vaccine which would help to protect potentially-exposed family members against developing Clostridial infection." Marshall added, "If this phase is telling us that live Clostridium germs are still present, then this is the time to use it. Even if the vaccine takes more than two weeks to give someone immunity, I think that dosing the well relatives of the affected may save us from some of those family member requiring treatment later, so we should proceed. We'll begin the vaccine shots on the contacts here tonight, and I would advise you to start immunizing family members in the hospital triage area as well."

"Just send it over and we'll get it started," Raines complied. "What about John Q. Citizen who walks in off the street and wants the shot?"

"I think we'd better limit it to family members for now," said Marshall, "since we only have enough vaccine to cover around twenty percent of the city's population."

Raines promised to keep him apprised of the numbers of ill planned for transport to the Convention Center and hung up with a deep feeling of foreboding.

Through the early morning hours, Raines walked the emergency department halls and pulled the next charts from the rack. He strode purposefully toward the gurneys parked in the hall, each containing at least one of the ill, but some gurneys now seating two family members experiencing diarrhea, weakness and fever. Most of these sick individuals also had concerned family members standing at the bedside.

Christie Fellows hung the antibiotic drips after medicating Mandy McConnell's nausea, pain, and fever. Mandy watched intently. Christy's expert reach to the overhead intravenous hook spoke of her experience and efficiency.

"I'm a nursing student at Jefferson," Mandy volunteered. "I hope I'll be as good as you are, someday."

"We really need you in nursing," responded Christy. "How are you feeling?"

Mandy shrugged but looked clearly concerned.

"The nausea is gone," Mandy said, "but I still have belly cramps, and I'm having trouble moving my fingers that I didn't have before."

Christie examined the young woman's forearms and hands and rapidly returned her eyes to the reassuring figure of 98% saturation on the oxygen monitor. Although Mandy was still breathing well, the hand weakness was a bad sign.

～

Raines dejectedly exited the resuscitation bay as the code team returned to their usual duties. A wife and mother in her thirties would not be returning home to her family. He walked to the family conference room to give the husband the bad news.

"I'm sorry, Mr. Meriwether, but we couldn't save her," he said simply. He knew that now was not the time for a detailed explanation of the resuscitation attempt.

"But we have children ...you've just *got* to help her!" McDonald pleaded, though Raines tried to tactfully bring him to the realization that the time for living with his thirty-two-year-old wife had ended. He was now a single parent after less than two hours of his wife's illness.

"I'm very sorry," Dr. Raines said simply. He had spoken the same shocking words to six families over the early morning hours of September 15. There was no easy way to give people information that would change their lives—information that their loved one was gone, and that there was nothing that could bring them back.

"But I just need to talk to her!" Meriwether panted.

Raines left the sobbing man in the comfort of a volunteer from the chaplain's office.

By four a.m., Mandy McConnell knew she was in trouble. Her hands had not moved for almost an hour, and each breath became an arduous task with no guarantee of its completion. Christie circled Mandy's gurney, testing her muscle function and watching the slide in her oxygen saturation levels from the desired 100% to a frightening mid-80's percentage.

"Dr. R.," she called into the hall, "she needs help."

Raines entered the room, knowing full well that they had preserved Mr. McConnell's distance from his worst nightmare for as long as possible. The fatigued father stood by the bedside, taking each breath with Mandy and praying for improvement that did not come.

"Mandy," Raines tenderly explained, "we need to help you to sleep while we breathe for you until you are stronger. Do you understand?"

Mandy, the only remaining light in the life of her father, remained stoic and even attempted a smile and nod.

"Prep twenty of etomidate for sedation," Raines instructed Christie. "I don't think we'll need the muscle relaxers for the intubation."

He stood at the head of Mandy's gurney and began to pre-oxygenate her with an Ambu bag and mask. Christie pushed the sedative medication as the respiratory therapist readied the equipment.

Raines slid the Macintosh blade into Mandy's weakened mouth and visualized her vocal cords. He pushed the endotracheal tube into position and began to force life-giving oxygen into Mandy's tired lungs.

Christie watched the oxygen saturation climb from 88 to 96 percent and patted Mr. McConnell's arm.

"She's safe now," the nurse reassured him.

"Call EMS, and move her to the Crisis Center," Raines directed. "They have a few more antitoxin patients off ventilatory support there now, and maybe we can get a vent."

McConnell stared down at his frail young daughter, the daughter whose friends, music, and laughter now seemed so far away. He just could not lose her, because there was nothing else left.

Raines needed to shore up McConnell's hope for the long haul.

"Mr. McConnell," he said quietly, "we'll have more antitoxin available in a few hours, and Dr. Mateo and Dr. Marshall at the Convention Center have found it effective in reversing the breathing problems. She is loaded with infection-fighting meds, and we will all be watching her closely."

"She'll be in good hands, and all we can do now is pray," Christie added.

McConnell nodded numbly and watched as the respiratory therapist's gentle squeeze on the plastic bag kept his little girl alive.

～

"Al, it's getting worse," said Raines quietly into the phone after paging Dr. Marshall at six a.m. "We've been seeing twenty new botulism cases an hour for the last two hours, and a lot more people are headed your way."

At least in Afghanistan, when things got bad ... even when that platoon of Afghan soldiers wandered onto a land mine, there was always an end in sight, Raines thought. At this point, the light at the end of the tunnel seemed to be from an oncoming train.

~

Christy Fellows had never before felt overwhelmed as a nurse. Even with the antibiotic drugs, the disease seemed to progress.

Christie looked down at the clipboard that listed the patients who were next to depart for the Crisis Center on a city bus commandeered by Slidell and the Philadelphia FEMA office.

"I've started the IV lines for this group of forty," she yelled to Karen, "and I'll start the paperwork for the next busload. We've got to have some supplies, and quick."

The hospital's overhead PX system blared.

"Code Five ... Morgue! Code Five ... Morgue! Code Five ... Morgue!"

Raines thought that this must truly be the strangest page that he had ever heard. Code Five was a security code, calling for the uniformed guards and the psychiatric staff to respond to an uncontrolled patient or visitor.

"Why would the morgue be the site of a security problem?" he muttered, with the answer then slamming him through his fatigue: the guy who demanded to talk to his dead wife.

Raines stacked his charts on the desk and called out to Dr. Richards.

"Chris, I'm responding to the code. I'll be back in a few minutes."

Raines jogged down the corridor to the stairs and then loped down the staircase two steps at a time, exiting in the hallway that led to the morgue. As he burst through into the hallway, he saw a small crowd gathered around the open morgue door.

"Drop the weapon, and exit the room!" commanded a guard, his service revolver cocked and pointing into the morgue.

The bystanders included two psychiatric orderlies and a psychiatric nurse, who remained flattened against the hallway wall to avoid gunfire. Behind the armed guard stood two more uniformed officers, each standing out of the view of the morgue door, and each with side arms drawn.

Raines could not see the source of the disturbance, but the culprit was apparently not planning to exit the room. He slipped in behind the armed guard at the door and stretched to look over the guard's shoulder.

Inside was Meriwether, the distraught father and former husband, standing in the center of the room with a nickel-plated revolver pressed against the right temple of forensic dentist Dr. Palmer Graves. Meriwether's eyes darted wildly about the room as he dragged Graves backward, away from the door.

Raines placed a hand on the guard's right shoulder ... the shoulder that held his service revolver and waited for a clear shot.

"Let me try; I know him," Raines said quietly, and stepped around the guard and into the morgue.

The gleam from the nickel revolver flashed across the doctor's face as Meriwether snapped it away from Graves's head and aimed at the center of Raines's chest.

"You have had terrible things happen to your family tonight," Raines began, "and none of us can possibly understand the depth of pain that you feel ... but we want to help. Your children need you now more than ever."

Meriwether kept the nickel-plated gun aimed at Raines, but he looked upward at the ceiling and began to cry.

"I just need to talk to her," he sobbed, "and they wouldn't

let me. They told me she's not here any longer, but I know she has to be here!"

"Just put down the gun and I promise we will find her," Raines said as he remembered his fruitless search for Aimee in that same strange room; a room strange to those still living due to its smells of formaldehyde and death.

"You'll help me find her?" asked Meriwether hopefully, relaxing his grip around Dr. Graves's neck.

"Yes, I promise that we will help you," said Raines with all the kindness that he could inject into his voice.

"You tried to help her when she got sick ...," Meriwether reasoned through the threads of sanity that remained.

"Yes, I tried," said Raines simply.

"I just need to talk to her," McDonald repeated as he lowered the revolver's barrel toward the floor.

The guard outside holstered his weapon, cautiously moved into the room next to Raines, and slowly reached for the gun in Meriwether's hand. The man, though pushed over the edge by fears and his burning desire for his family's stability, did not resist as the guard slipped the weapon from his hand and tucked it into his waistband.

"*Clear!*" reported the guard, and his uniformed colleagues rushed into the room. The three guards roughly seized Meriwether's arms, but then released them when Raines waved them off the grief-stricken man.

Raines spoke to him.

"We're going to go find your wife, just as I said, but first you need to take a little medication for your nerves."

"What kind of medication?" asked Meriwether. "Are you trying to kill me?"

"No, we're not trying to kill you," Raines smiled. "The medication is a mild sedative called lorazepam, and it will help you begin planning to get back home to your children."

"Okay," agreed a resigned Meriwether.

The psychiatric nurse stepped forward and treated the

trembling man's right biceps to the injection. Meriwether sat down as Raines asked one of the guards to attempt to find Mrs. Meriwether. The guard stepped from the morgue and headed for the loading dock exit.

Raines sat beside Meriwether and looked at Dr. Graves, who was deeply pallid and mopping his aristocratic brow.

"Are you okay, Doctor?" asked Raines.

"Yes … Oh my, yes. I fear that I've just worked a bit too late tonight!" said the old dentist truthfully.

Chapter 29

TRIAGE

Pennsylvania Convention Center; 15 September 2008

Nah, I never eat at home," replied the teenager.
The young man was the only family member of five who did not exhibit the fever, weakness, and diarrhea of the super germ. His work at Burger King provided him alternate dining opportunities, and, in the opinion of DMAT family physician Dr. Jillian Case, protected him from the spread of the infection that began at a family mealtime. She made a note for the Philadelphia Department of Public Health to screen the family's cookware and eating utensils with one of the Marine SMART membranes.

The NJ-1 Disaster Medical Assistance Team's triage tent bulged with another forty or fifty patients to be seen, but they were all "green tagged," thus the team could sort through them without moving into an emergent mode to stabilize urgent breathing problems. The patients had entered the DMAT complex through the decontamination tent, where they were registered, rinsed, placed in a paper gown and given a disposable blanket. The Marine decon team complained that it did little good to wash the outside of someone whose problem was inside, but Major Tower pointed out, in typical blunt Marine Corps fashion, their responsibility to halt the possible spread of infection from a patient's skin.

The Disaster Mortuary Assistance Team pathologists received the few patients who were deceased upon arrival, and the Disaster Medical Assistance Team paramedics triaged the living. Those patients with breathing problems or the inability to stand were "red tagged" in triage and moved to the head of the treatment line. The triage team established intravenous lines on the ill patients, but no antibiotics or antitoxins were given in the tent because of the waning supply.

The portable toilet area behind the decon tent smelled of illness and death. Marines in containment suits collected red plastic bags of clothing from fifty-five gallon drums labeled "Contaminated Waste" and transported them for processing. Although this was an unpopular duty, the Marines dutifully suited up and reported for their shifts.

"Hell, John," said Dr. Case quietly to chief nurse John Harrell. "Are we really accomplishing anything with the IV lines? Until we get more antitoxin from Sanofi-Pasteur, there's nothing to give them that makes any difference!"

"At least we'll have the patient hydrated and the IV access when the additional stuff comes in," said Harrell.

"By the end of a twelve-hour triage shift," Case admitted, "I'm so frustrated, I could chew nails. I lie awake and look at the roof of the sleep tent all night."

"It will get better when we get the tools, Jill," said Harrell. "We've just got to hold on till then."

~

Dr. Palmer Grace had little challenge in cataloguing the dead in Philadelphia. Almost all had identification in their pockets and frightened family members to verify who they had been in life. The DMORT's two pathologists signed death certificates in stacks of twenty-five to simplify the count. An employee of the county clerk's office, the DMORT, and the Red Cross all recorded the names of the deceased to ensure that the "final disposition" was correct. The refrigeration trucks remained in service, with their contents of human firewood stacked high enough that there were no plans for individual funerals.

One unidentified body interested Dr. Grace. A middle-aged drunk found near the river in a decrepit train yard proved to have no identification and no family members to identify the body. Dr. Grace did an online search for dental records and found a match with the Armed Forces Institute of Pathology.

Robert Walker had been a Vietnam-era serviceman, and the Department of Defense database address in Minnesota was over twenty-five years old. Grace even did a Google search for the wife listed as his legal next of kin, but had no luck in finding her. The long road for Fuzzy Walker had ended, and his internationally known concert pianist daughter would never even know his resting place.

Chapter 30

TOLLS

Virginia; 15 September 2008

"N ot him!" yelled Landrum. He hit the speed-dial number for Taylor's cell phone.

"He just filled up with a credit card in Harrisonburg, Virginia," said Landrum, fingering the map of Interstate 81 leading to the southwest across the state of Virginia. "In two more hours, he'll be in Tennessee."

"Like hell he will!" assured Taylor. "We're refueling in Charlottesville, and then we'll head north for the intercept."

~

Ali Zarif heard the helicopter before he saw it, and was already checking the Palm's map for an earlier exit for a cross-country route. The GPS chip in the handheld told Zarif that he was near the town of Staunton, Virginia.

Just as the Bell 201 became visible on the horizon, Zarif turned onto state highway 250 and sped west toward the Spruce Knob National Recreation Area. He slowed to sixty as he entered the small town of Liberty, Virginia.

"He just exited and is headed west on a state road toward a small town— ironically its name is Liberty, Virginia," Taylor reported to Landrum as he dropped the binoculars back into the Bell's door pocket.

"We have two trooper units approaching the area, and we'll contact the local police department to get their ground units moving. Take him down," commanded Landrum. "Too much chance of losing him for good off of the interstate."

Ali Zarif, entering an older commercial area of Liberty and without benefit of a rearview mirror, did not see the Virginia state trooper until the car pulled along side his Buick and turned on its blue lights.

Lights flashing, the trooper was prepared with a 12-gauge riot gun lying on the passenger seat. The second trooper vehicle pulled in behind Zarif, and a Liberty Police Department vehicle joined the pursuit as well.

"Nowhere to run," decided Zarif. "It is Allah's time now."

Zarif pulled the Buick into the parking area of a road-side truck stop, advancing until the front bumper was inches from the restaurant's peeling, concrete-block walls. He calmly remained behind the wheel of the vehicle, lowering the driver's side window and awaiting the inevitable, unpleasant encounter with the Virginia law officers.

Senior trooper Reynolds exited his cruiser, riot gun in hand, as the remaining Virginia trooper vehicle and the Liberty PD unit boxed in the Buick. The Liberty Police unit added its rotating beacons of command to the parking area, now awash in a sea of blue strobes. The two officers behind the Buick exited with handguns drawn, taking cover behind their vehicle doors and fixing aim on the figure behind the wheel of the burgundy vehicle. This adjustment of their positions behind the police cruiser doors was life saving unless the suspect fired armor-piercing rounds.

"Hands on the wheel!" commanded Trooper Reynolds, with the twelve-gauge leveled at Zarif's head. "Do not attempt to move!"

Zarif looked at the old building in front of him, noting its peeling paint and the layer of dust on the lower edges of its metallic window frames. He heard the distant rumble of the big truck diesel engines in the rear parking lot and the cackling laughter of a "truck stop honey."

As the trooper approached the Buick, Zarif stared straight ahead, deeply concentrating on his prayer. When the officer had closed to three feet, Zarif quietly ended with "Allah Akbar" and pressed the radio-frequency detonator.

The two explosive jackets located in the rear seat of the Buick ignited simultaneously, instantly incinerating Zarif's car plus the vehicle of Trooper Reynolds. Although meant for suicide bombers, the kilogram of Semtex in each jacket was effective in turning the Buick into a hand grenade, blowing metal and glass through the police cars behind as though they were made of paper. The concrete walls and front glass of the restaurant became fatal projectiles, blowing through patrons unlucky enough to be enjoying the truckers' fare in the front half of the restaurant. Reynolds died instantly, as did one of the officers providing cover from behind a police car door.

Smoldering carnage and eerie silence were the only remnants of the blast, slowly followed by the moans of the injured on the restaurant floor.

"Operations Center, we have a situation!" reported Taylor from the chopper. "We have a major explosive event from the suspect vehicle ... Request available ambulance and fire response to coordinates 382640 North by 0785244 West!"

"Damn!" spat Landrum. "They're still adding to the toll!"

Chapter 31

FROM ASHES

The computer was a bit smoked, as you can see," reported the National Security Agency's resident computer guru. "However, we pulled the hard drive and found it undamaged. He reformatted the disc, of course, but using our recovery software followed by some work on the encryption, we were able to retrieve most of the information. There is some possibility of an error with the first letter of each e-mail name, but overall, we expect an 80 percent recovery of data."

The Green Building's conference room was silent as the FBI agents digested the possibility of adding dozens of Middle Eastern and American names to their lists of likely terrorists.

"How many e-mail names did you come up with?" inquired Special Agent in Charge Wells.

"Around three hundred," the NSA geek said.

"We still have thousands of e-mails to sort through," reported Landrum, "but we've already identified several priority targets for investigation."

"Go on," requested Wells.

Landrum stepped to the head of the table, where a digital projector was aimed at a clean white wall. He plugged his laptop into the projector and paged through the digital photo directories stored on the unit's hard drive. He selected the "Zarif" picture directory and hit the "Enter" key. A digital photo of the destroyed Liberty truck stop flashed into view on the wall.

"Dr. Zarif's car contained two explosive jackets, each carrying around a kilo of Semtex plastic explosive. The Czech government added ethylene glycol dinitrate to the Semtex formulation after the PanAm 103 attack, in an attempt to make the compound more detectable by its smell. This formulation was missing the EGD odor agent, but there are still over two hundred international sources of the explosive type used.

"With the explosion," Landrum went on, "Zarif left behind only a charred AK-74 assault rifle, a 9mm pistol, and the spiral wire binding of a notebook of some kind."

He clicked the next slide to show the remnants of the Buick, with the incinerated Texas State Trooper cruiser crushed beside it.

"There were no recoverable fragments of paper, and the cell phone in the vehicle was turned into a mound of melted silicon. The death toll for the explosion was fourteen and another thirty-six were injured. Regardless, it appears that the suspect was headed southwest toward Tennessee when his trip ended prematurely."

"So, where was he going?" prodded Wells.

Landrum referred the inch thick sheaf of papers that he held in his left hand.

"One indicator may be the NSA cell phone call intercept from the afternoon after the Philadelphia attack. At 10:20 a.m., Zarif placed a call to a cell phone registered to the Delaware Bay Benevolence Fund, with conversation as follows:

"Zarif: 'The early reports are favorable ... What is your progress?'

"Unknown on cell phone: 'We are between Knoxville and Birmingham and expect to be within the destination by morning prayers. What of Musa?'

"Zarif: 'He will sleep with the container.'

"The call lasted for three and a half minutes.

"The NSA also found an e-mail on the torched hard drive from Zarif to an imam. The recipient is apparently located at a mosque in Houston. The e-mail noted that 'Faithful Travelers' would be arriving and requested assistance during their stay.

Landrum looked at Agent in Charge Wells's craggy face, concerned that his deductions on the destination of the perpetrators would be considered too circumstantial— just a plain wild guess.

"We theorize that an unknown number of accomplices transported the attack truck with a shipping container through Tennessee and Alabama and continued into Texas on the 11th of September," summarized Landrum. "For their destination to be reached 'by morning prayers' would place them within ten or eleven hours of Knoxville, and the location may well be the Bilal Center mosque in Houston, Texas.

"We think that 'Musa' refers to a member of the Al-Douri mosque, Musa Alamoudi, a twenty-six-year-old electronics salesman," Landrum continued. "We've attempted to locate Mr. Alamoudi, but he was absent from both his job and his South Philadelphia apartment. We would like to press for surveillance on the Houston mosque and attempt to identify the accomplices that remain alive.

"In addition, we have obtained the blue 1994 International truck's vehicle identification number from the

Landers Trucking Company of Phoenix," Landrum said, "and have issued state and national Suspect Vehicle Searches in Tennessee, Alabama, Mississippi, Louisiana, and Texas, in order to locate it as soon as possible.

"We also uncovered on the computer's hard drive Zarif's request for the pumping station weapons from contacts located in the Middle East. There were eight AK's requested, and with one suspect dying in Philadelphia, one in New York and one in Virginia; plus the two in custody in New York, that leaves three rifle-holders who may still in the land of the living. Our team has questioned the two men in custody in New York, but they are not talking. We have no guesses as to whether all three remaining suspects relocated to Texas after the attack.

"We'll need Texas State Trooper and Texas Bureau of Investigation assists," directed Wells, "and we'll send a team of four to Houston. We will also need to fly the men in custody in New York to Quantico for a little more in-depth discussion.

"We have discovered a rental agreement for a meat-packing warehouse with the Delaware Bay Benevolence Fund providing the money, but the lease signed by a company called Biolimit," Landrum added.

"More importantly," he related with pride, "we have recovered from Zarif's hard drive several e-mails of interest from someone calling himself 'Khalid.' These e-mails include discussion of a 'product delivery' and a 'shipping schedule.'

"If 'Khalid' is the origin of the toxin, there are international implications, because the e-mails originated in Iran."

"Iran … Oh hell!" said Wells aloud. "I'll need a printout of all of the 'Khalid' e-mails and the NSA's best information on the origin of the emails."

Wells was a veteran G-man and was too familiar with the problems involved with threading through the bureaucratic nightmare and placing important information on a senior desk. Even with internationally significant information, he expected the wheels to turn slowly.

"I'll forward the Iranian e-mail copies to the Terrorist Threat Center and call the FBI Counterterrorism Division. The FBI Director needs to be in on this by tonight ... and the State Department ... and even the White House."

"There's more that they're going to want to know, Chief," reported Landrum. "The financial records on the hard drive confirm what we got from the bank. Large amounts of money flowed from offshore accounts through the Al-Douri Mosque and directly into the Delaware Bay Fund. Major funding sources include the Brotherhood of Islamic Jihad, which is primarily based in Algeria, but also with a large presence in Egypt.

"The largest amount of money came from the Muslim Liberation Front, based in Syria," he added. "This thing has 'international event' and 'United Nations involvement' stamped all over it."

Landrum paused for effect.

"They were also getting money from Harvard University and both the state of Pennsylvania and the U.S government, so I would expect a rodeo of political ass-covering. The big boys in the Bureau are definitely gonna want in on this one early."

Wells scratched his head with concern as he thought of the political fallout for the Bureau when the press got wind that the FBI was pointing out governmental contributions to terrorism.

"We also need the info on the investigation of the remainder of the Al-Douri leaders who are still in Philadelphia," Wells added. "We don't know if additional people had knowledge of the attack. We'll also need a rundown on names and locations of the foreign organizations sending money to the Benevolence Fund that are known to have principal players residing in the United States," Wells concluded.

It was all about to hit the fan.

Chapter 32

COVERT OPS

Langley, Virginia; 15 September 2008

Talbot walked briskly through Washington's Reagan Airport, carrying only a second rumpled suit in a worn carry-on bag. He hurried through the entrance to meet a gray Crown Victoria waiting outside.

"We need you to brief the Deputy Director on the current sit-rep in Philadelphia," said Senior Agent McInnis. "Then we'll get you back out on the 20:15 plane."

Talbot nodded, much too experienced to ask any more questions in an unsecured environment.

～

"Talbot," he said at the Langley security checkpoint, and he placed his right index finger on the laser screen for identification. He followed McInnis through the double-blast doors and into the secure conference room. He recognized the CIA Deputy Director for Operations, Sidney Green, at the end of the conference table, but did not know the other three men in the room.

"Please start us off," Mcinnis nodded to Talbot.

The rumpled man rose, cleared his throat, and began the story of the messy situation in Philly.

"The attack was initiated by a group of Islamic fundamentalists, funded by a group titled the Delaware Bay Benevolence Fund, which has ties to the Brotherhood for Islamic Jihad and the Muslim Liberation Front," Talbert summarized.

"Dr. Ali Zarif, a Philadelphia computer science professor, and at least seven accomplices backed a truck and shipping container into a Philadelphia water department pumping station, dispatched the station's three workers and a guard, then introduced botulinum toxin and possibly Clostridium germs into the water supply. The toxin in the water supply killed an initial eight hundred people, and another thousand are currently ill but still surviving.

"Over the last twelve hours, a second wave of botulism has occurred," Talbot continued, "with the disease less severe, but apparently actively infectious and capable of being spread to others through diarrhea fluid and close personal contact. The source of the bacteria and toxin appears to be Dr. Khalid Atoomb, an Iraqi microbiologist working in Tehran at an unknown location.

"The Clostridium germs causing the second wave of botulism have not yet been recovered," said Talbot, "but the fevers and diarrhea seem to be resistant to all of the antibiotic therapies tried. Botulism antitoxin is working to get some of the ill off ventilators, but the supply from the manufacturer is limited and the strategic national stock nearly depleted. There is a plan to vaccinate the family contacts of the toxin-affected against the Clostridium germs, but results will take at least two weeks and there is only enough of the immunization to cover five percent of the Philadelphia population."

The mood in the conference room was somber.

McInnis stood and pushed the button on a laser pointer that slid open a large digital screen on the wall to the right of the conference table. He advanced the slides and presented the group a photo of an Arab man still in graduate school at the time of the photograph.

"Dr. Khalid Atoomb," said McInnis, "thirty-two, an Iraqi national with training in engineering and microbiology here in the United States. He is apparently working under the direction of the Iranian government at an unknown location in Tehran, and is thought to be the source of the infectious agent based on his training in gene splicing and his e-mail traffic with Dr. Zarif. The NSA recovered an e-mail from a computer hard drive belonging to the late Dr. Zarif, and 'Khalid' notes 'shipping dates' in August of approximately two thousand liters of a 'product.' We have found no transatlantic shipping of containers from Iran to the Port of Philadelphia during August or early September. However, more than 170,000 containers were unloaded from international ships in the Port of Philadelphia during this period.

"Although the laboratory site is unknown, we know the location of Dr. Atoomb's residence in western Tehran, and the apartment is under observation by our Tehran station chief. We have the financial trails of a large amount of funding that was funneled through the Philadelphia group and records of the arms and truck purchases by Dr. Zarif with these funds." McInnis then awaited the deputy director's comments.

"Thank you, Mr. McInnis," said Green, "and thank you for making the trip, Agent Talbot. We will be following closely your reports from Philadelphia."

After McInnis and Talbot left the secure conference room, the muscular man with the steel-gray hair, who sat quietly on the deputy director's right, patiently awaited guidance to speak.

"So how do you propose we talk with Dr. Atoomb, Charlie?" asked Green.

"Sir," briefed ex-Delta Force Lieutenant Colonel Charles Stroud, chief of the Special Activities Division, "the operation we recommend utilizes six of our Special Activities staff, flown via Aero Contractors, Ltd., to Incirclik for staging. We plan to depart Turkey by Russian MI-17 helicopter, approach over the Caspian Sea and secure this location eighteen miles inland in the Chalus River Gorge of the Elburz Mountains."

Stroud tapped the icon for a digital photo on his laptop, which his secure wireless computer system placed on the viewing screen in front of the director. The image was a satellite shot that revealed a high-altitude view of the rugged Iranian mountains on the southern shore of the Caspian Sea. Stroud's second click zoomed the satellite image in for a detailed view of the Chalus Gorge, already covered by snow in the photo that was taken on the morning of September 15.

"Our four Agency men in Tehran will preposition a van on this rural road," Stroud said as he advanced to the next image, "and will then hold the subject under observation on the night of the snatch."

He advanced the images yet again, and the group saw a digital photo of a sunlit, older apartment building located on the western border of the city of Tehran.

"The subject lives on the second floor of this housing project," he continued, "in a corner apartment with an elderly woman living next door."

The next digital photo, taken with a telephoto lens, showed the partially hidden face of Atoomb's sparsely toothed, and apparently shy, Iranian neighbor.

"We will make the snatch," Stroud reported confidently, "and depart by van for the Elburz Mountain site. We will return via the Caspian, refueling in Azerbaijan, and interrogate the subject on the return flight."

"If we are compromised," Stroud continued, "the evasion

and escape plan will include a second chopper twenty-four hours later, and a rendezvous for extraction in this plain to the southeast of Rasht, Iran." Stroud's final image revealed a low, grassy plain surrounded by snowy mountain peaks.

The spec-ops colonel concluded: "We anticipate the capture could be made on September 18, if approved by the director."

"What is our current inventory of the Soviet helos?" asked Deputy Director Green.

"We have three MI-17's and an MI-8. They are now armed with our own HELLFIRE missiles and 20mm chain guns. The best thing about the Ruskie chopper, other than it fitting into the Caspian, is that it flies just as well on one engine as it does on two."

Green turned to the small, mustachioed man seated to Stroud's right.

"Anything to add, Lopez?"

"Nothing, sir."

"Geek?" inquired Green.

"Nothing to add, Mr. Director," replied the frail-looking man with the horn-rimmed glasses.

"You have a tentative go on the op," Green authorized. "The point of no return will be 2200 hours, Zulu, on the 17th."

"Yes, sir," nodded Stroud as he confirmed that the "Top Secret/Director's Eyes Only" digital images were returned to the computer's "Atoomb Rendition" operation directory and secured with his pass code. He then placed the laptop in an aluminum briefcase that he locked and placed in front of his chair.

Chapter 33

EPIDEMIC

Philadelphia; 15-16 September 2008

Dr. Tony Mateo, just after beginning his evening shift, stood with Dr. Marshall and accepted the responsibility for the Crisis Center patients. At Mandy McConnell's bedside, near the right wall of the Convention Center's care area, things were going poorly. Her blood pressure spiraled progressively lower and her pulses were fainter. Mateo asked the DMAT nurse working this section of the care area to begin five micrograms per minute of dopamine in an attempt to stimulate her blood pressure and salvage her life.

Matthew McConnell stood before the two physicians near Mandy's bedside and listened to the horrid truth he already knew about her prognosis. Lost in concern for his daughter's life, he seemed hesitant to bring up the foreboding truth about himself.

"I started having diarrhea this morning, doctor," McConnell admitted, "but I didn't want to leave Mandy. Now my face feels funny, and I can't see well."

Al Marshall looked deep into the face of the tortured man. McConnell's goal had simply been to save his daughter's life, and now his was in jeopardy as well.

As Marshall turned, he wondered how many of the huddled family members had also been secretly hiding the spread of the infection, and whether he could get the results of the blood and stool cultures quickly enough to identify the germ, select the proper antibiotic and head off an overwhelming epidemic.

~

Over the morning hours, Christie had started dozens of intravenous lines, initiated weakness evaluations on more than two hundred patients, and lost track of how many ambulances and buses had departed for the Crisis Center. The emergency room team gave a combination of oral antibiotics to anyone who could tolerate medication by mouth, and intravenous antibiotics to those who could not. Now the hospital's supply of ciprofloxacin was depleted, and they were dangerously low on sulfa drugs and gentamicin. Even with all of the antimicrobial drugs tried, the fever and diarrhea of the infection seemed to progress.

"Dr. R.," she noted with resigned fatigue, "all the cases of fluid they brought up from central supply are gone. I'm not sure what else to do except to pat hands!"

Christie was good at patting hands, because she was a caring nurse who was more interested in her patients' needs than in their paperwork and nursing care plans.

"We have problems, Al," Raines said quietly into the phone. "Over the last three hours, we have been seeing sixty new botulism infections an hour. We're basically out of antibiotics and about to run out of IV fluids."

"We'll try to call in a few favors, Ron," Marshall said with resignation.

The Michigan Department of Health was sending more botulinum vaccine, and the last of the Sanofi-Pasteur antitoxin in existence was in a truck speeding toward the Pennsylvania Convention Center.

As Marshall was about to depart for the evening, he played the desperation card. "Sorry to have to ask, Tony, but we're almost out of everything that we need for this infection phase. Could you call in any favors from military channels?"

"Sure, no problem," the old doctor grinned. "I'll call the naval hospitals in Norfolk and Bethesda."

"At least the families will think we're doing something for them," Marshall said dejectedly.

The death toll for the second wave now stood at four hundred, and the Convention Center was stacked with more than a thousand people with diarrhea and muscle weakness. All of the strategic national stock ventilators were in use, and another three hundred people supported their family members with Ambu bags. To halt the spread of infection in the Crisis Center, the Center caregivers now followed Tony Mateo's simple but effective plan. The thousands with diarrhea used red plastic bags, which the Marines collected while wearing class B containment suits. Since the center had no source for radiation treatment of the bags of fluid, the Marines packed them into a bank of microwaves for processing before they were loaded into a dumpster. The SMART membranes' screens indicated that after "nuking" the deadly fluid, no traces of the botulinum toxin remained.

Mateo looked at the throng of the ill and their hovering family members.

"We can put more people in here, but I don't know who will even have time to look at them," he said to Marshall. "Everybody has been on twenty-four-hour operations for five days, and we're going to see people die because there is simply no one to squeeze an Ambu bag for them."

"I'm not looking forward to telling Raines that Mandy McConnell died today," admitted Marshall. "Her father's a wreck and sick with the infection on top of it. He told me he doesn't want to get any better."

Mateo reassured him.

"We'll have antibiotics, fluids, and IV sets from Naval Hospital Norfolk and from Bethesda," Mateo said. "But it'll take eight or ten hours to package and fly it in."

Alphonse Marshall wondered if he were the right man to lead the search for relief from an infectious problem that seemed to have no solution. He had grown up in a working man's household in Alabama and never planned to be at the head of the most advanced medical research organization in the world and its attempt to head off the worst infectious nightmare since the Great Plague. He considered calling in help from Atlanta but knew what his fellow infectious disease doctors would ask: "What about the cultures? What about the antibiotic sensitivity testing?"

The information just was not yet available.

～

Dr. Ron Raines sank with fatigue into a chair in the emergency department's dictation alcove.

There nothing I can do to make this any better, he thought. *aren't working, and the sick and dying are still streaming in the door.*

He rubbed a hand over his burning eyes and wondered if the disaster would simply die out in Philadelphia or spread to other cities as desperate people tried to escape the infected city. Already, a case had appeared in New York and another in Atlanta in people who felt well when boarding airplanes in Philadelphia.

He looked up to see Christy's eyes focused directly on his face. She looked down quickly and then looked up at Raines again to see if he had spotted her.

Wonder what that was all about? thought Raines. *Probably found something I did wrong ... or she just knows I cannot do a damn thing to help these people.*

In thirty-eight years of challenges, Raines had never felt like hiding from a problem—but he felt like it now.

~

"Hey, my wife needs some-a that IV stuff, too!" exploded a thin, scruffy man wearing a Lynard Skynard T-shirt.

At almost seven in the morning on September 16, Marshall returned to relieve Mateo from Crisis Center responsibility, but fatigue and stress was taking its toll on patients and family members as well.

"Sir, we'll have more IV fluids and antibiotics in just an hour or so," Marshall tried to pacify him.

"You think just because you're the big, important black guy in charge, you can treat the white people like second-class citizens!" responded Scruffy.

A still neatly pressed Navy battle dress uniform entered the conversation, the eagles on the collar reinforcing a long-term habit of handling problems.

"Sir," Mateo said to the outraged man, "I'm feeling calm today, so I'm going to give you the opportunity to sit down and shut the hell up."

Scruffy sat.

Marshall looked at the crusty old captain who glowered at the man like an old bulldog: growing a bit slower on the hunt, but still baring significant teeth.

"I'm getting too old for this," Mateo quietly confided to Marshall. The Navy doctors had advised the captain to retire years before, after he had suffered a heart attack and undergone a coronary bypass. Now, his morning regimen included taking three heart pills and an arthritis medicine.

"Thanks, Tony," said Marshall, convinced that he couldn't feel much lower.

Just as the team was assembling for shift change report, the Convention Center air was pierced by the shriek of Marshall's pager. He anxiously dialed the 412 area code number and received an answer on the first ring.

"Marshall, answering a page," he said.

"Yes, Dr. Marshall, this is Dr. Herb Stallings, the state lab's director. I came in early to read your cultures, and I'm afraid I have something I just don't understand. We confirmed the presence of large amounts of botulinum toxin A, but we're finding no evidence of Clostridium germs. We do, however, have growth of almost pure cultures of Enterobacter germs!"

"Enterobacter?" puzzled Marshall. "Are you sure? How could an Enterobacter be the toxin producer?"

Then it all became painfully clear.

"It's a hybrid!" Marshall exclaimed. "This germ is genetically engineered with botulinum toxin placed in a carrier organism ... and there are only two places on earth where it could have happened: the biowarfare defense laboratories of the United States and the biologic weapons program of the former Soviet Union."

"That level of microbiology is way over my head," remarked Stallings. "I'll call you back when we have the Enterobacter germ's antibiotic sensitivities in another two to three days."

Across the expansive floor of the Pennsylvania Convention Center, the doors opened, and a coffee-stained truck driver entered wearing a Sanofi-Pasteur jacket and a two-day growth of beard. He seemed shocked at the maze of human life support around him and looked around for someone who might be in charge.

"That must be our factory representative," Marshall said as he began to cross the floor in anticipation.

"I'm from Sanofi-Pasteur," the haggard driver reported when Marshall reached him. "We drove nonstop from the Swiftwater lab and got here as soon as we could. You got some unloading help for the antitoxin?"

"Sure," responded Marshall. "We got the whole Marine Corps!"

~

At her Jefferson emergency room triage desk around six a.m., Karen Winslow felt it first in the lower abdomen, a peculiar cramping subtly signaling a problem. She had no diarrhea, but maybe that was because there was no time to entertain such nuisances. She thought she should leave her triage post since she might be infectious, but there simply was no one else with the experience to meet the deluge of new patients. She decided to tell Dr. Raines at the end of the shift … just one more hour.

By seven a.m., Karen felt as though her arms and legs were made of lead, and she was beginning to see double as her eyelids and the intricate muscles controlling her eye movement began to fail. She could no longer keep the infection a secret. She knew that she belonged in the Crisis Center, along with the thousand who hoped for a magical recovery.

Karen had difficulty reaching the locker with the stethoscope in her right hand. She left her purse inside and closed the door, using all of her determination to snap the padlock closed. Suddenly, the room seemed to tilt at a crazy angle, and she found herself lying on the cool, dark tile of the locker room floor. Only inches in front of her eyes was the light green tile of the emergency department walls, a tile she knew so well, though her eyes now focused poorly.

She knew intimately the green tile that had stood solidly behind her as she had suffered through eighteen years of trials and tribulations with the patients of Jefferson. As she took her last breath, her thoughts were of her husband— and whether he would be able to care for their daughters alone.

Chapter 34

HEALTHY LIFE

Martha's Vineyard; 28 September 2008

Delayne Worchester took the bundle of mail and dropped in on the table in the sunroom. The Vineyard's morning sun poured through the skylights, helping her forget the fall chill in the air. She pushed aside the bills and selected two of the new magazines to enjoy during her bath.

With curiosity, she noticed the manila envelope from "The Publishers of *Healthy Life*" and opened it, expecting yet another offer for a book on organic gardening or isometric exercises. Instead, the envelope contained a pair of gold foil packets, with "Longevity Tea" emblazoned on the front. She looked again at the envelope and noticed that the publisher had misspelled her name as "Delaine," just as it did when she received the magazine.

She turned over the foil packet to read the ingredients:

"a blend of imported Turkish teas, vitamins A, B1, B6, B12, C, and E, plus antioxidants for reversal of the aging process." The tea had no carbs or fat grams.

Hmm, sounds good, she thought as she filled the teapot and put in on the stove to warm. She then took her pair of magazines and entered the bathroom for a leisurely soak.

The telephone in the sunroom shattered the quiet of the near-perfect morning.

"Oh, bother ..." grumped Delayne from her warm, sudsy cocoon, "You'll just have to call back."

She returned to her article on the diet of wild birds in the Atlantic northeast.

Chapter 35

PREPS

Camp Peary, Virginia; 15 September 2008

The white Gulfstream V taxied down Camp Peary's Runway 23, effortlessly lifted off, and banked over the Atlantic. The runway was restricted, technically a part of the Navy's Armed Forces Experimental Training Center, but the new CIA trainee dormitories nearby revealed the truth and the ongoing use of the training center for OGA activities. Nosy neighbors in Williamsburg were simply told that the activities at Camp Peary were classified issues of national security.

Charlie Stroud looked over his handpicked Special Activities team as would the proud father of an all-American athlete. Each was dressed casually in warm ski clothing and had at his feet the particular combination of footlocker/briefcase/backpack that he had found most useful over the years of deployment. None of the backpacks was of military issue, and the group could have easily passed for tourists, businessmen, or even graduate students.

Stroud thought that the grad student similarity was particularly appropriate, since four of the men did carry graduate degrees, three were proficient in Arabic, and two even spoke Farsi.

They were a bit heavily armed for students, however; most were equipped with a repeatedly cleaned Heckler and Koch silenced MP-5SD3 submachine gun, and each carried his side arm of choice. Stroud smiled at the personality revealed in the handguns, which varied from a shiny, nickel-plated Ruger .357 snubnose carried by Wills to the basic black, nondescript Colt Commander .45 favored by Lopez.

Stroud had picked each of the men for the particular set of skills he brought to the party. Lopez, the quiet Hispanic, was a linguist and the team's medic, trained by Army Special Forces through the grueling two-year process to become an 18D. To graduate the 18D training program, he had to be proficient in the medical care and resuscitation of his special operations team members, plus have basic skills in dentistry and veterinary medicine. He had worked with Stroud in Delta Force and exhibited the judgment that always kept the team's safety in the foreground.

Becker, also a linguist, was trained by Special Forces and worked for Delta Force as an 18C, engineer sergeant. He was skilled in building things—but even more skilled in blowing them apart. Becker was bearded, quiet, and able to work with the explosives he found in any nation. His benign appearance belied the carnage that frequently followed his activities.

Wills, the youngest and most aggressive, was a twenty-six-year-old, redheaded fireplug of a man, a linguist and a veteran of SEAL Team Six. He still followed the SEAL training program's habit of firing at least a thousand training rounds a month; just to have the skills when he needed them. Stroud occasionally had trouble curtailing Wills's enthusiasm.

Thomas was even older than Stroud, a reliable, hard and brown grandfather clock of a man with a proud background as a Delta weapons expert. He was a graduate of the elite Army sniper school and routinely placed accurate rounds on target from two thousand yards with his chosen weapon, a vintage telescopic-sight M-14 rifle.

Then there was the Geek. He was the only man who had not been "sheep-dipped" from the military; his background included a Masters in electrical engineering from MIT. He functioned as the team's communication expert and was thought to be able to obtain a satellite link from a pair of cans and a string. The Geek's skinny, bespectacled appearance belied his ability to function, however, on a previous occasion he had proven himself capable of putting a round through an opponent's head when the team was in jeopardy.

Stroud watched as each specialist assured his readiness for his component of "the package," then took an Ambien and settled in to sleep as the team flew across the Atlantic. The men had long since forgotten rank, except for the courtesy "Colonel" that Stroud was afforded on the plane. Everywhere else, he was "Charlie," and even federal agents unknown to the team would find that for security reasons they were misdirected to an uninvolved party if they asked for the team's leader.

The five men of military background had made the switch to CIA Special Activities for several reasons. Sure, doubling one's salary was nice, and the deployments of two or three weeks beat the hell out of a yearlong deployment to Iraq. Free of military grooming regulations, two of the men wore beards and all had non-regulation haircuts. The most important reason for the move from the military was that each relished the opportunity to play on the "First Team," a team entrusted with the most important and the most sensitive issues of national security. The Geek had once remarked that he did not know of any other legal way to have so much fun.

They would refuel in Amsterdam and arrive at Incirclik Air Force Base, Turkey, during the afternoon of September 16th. After final preparations and a nod from the CIA command structure, they would initiate the mission.

Chapter 36

CST

Philadelphia; 16 September 2008

The incident command meeting convened at six p.m. Drs. Marshall, Mateo, Raines and Case were present, plus Slidell of FEMA, Graves of the Red Cross, Tower of the CBIRF, and the representatives of Philadelphia EMS and Police Department. As usual, a rumpled Talbot occupied the rear corner, but he now showed the fresh motivation handed down by his superiors in Washington. Krause reiterated the numbers of the dead and ill, the arrival of the desperately needed botulinum antitoxin supply, and the frighteningly progressive nature of the infectious phase of the mystery germ's spread in the population.

"One bright point for today is the arrival of additional military assistance," he added. "This is Captain Ledbetter of the New Jersey National Guard's 21st Weapons of Mass Destruction Civil Support Team. Captain, tell us about your unit."

A blonde man in his late twenties—wearing a battle dress uniform, glasses, and the crossed beakers of the Army's Chemical Corps branch—stood uneasily to face the group of tired public servants. He looked more like a violin student than a battle-hardened warrior.

"Gentlemen and lady," Captain Ledbetter began haltingly, "we are the New Jersey National Guard's 21st WMD-CST. I'd like to be able to tell you we are here to save the day, but I'm afraid that's not true."

A look of concern rapidly crossed the room.

"We were formed in 2001 and are a reserve sector unit of twenty-two individuals assigned to AGR positions—that is, full-time Active Guard and Reserve, each on a three-year tour to support catastrophes of biologic, chemical, and nuclear importance such as this. We were created, at least on paper, to have the capacity to decontaminate, carry sophisticated laboratory equipment for the identification of chemicals and pathogens, and be staffed with a nuclear safety officer and a physician.

"The truth of our federal and state funding is, unfortunately, that none of the nation's thirty-two WMD-CST's are now provided with the planned MALS van for laboratory testing, and only one has a nuclear science officer. We have a physician's assistant, not a nuclear-biologic-chemical physician, and we now carry Motrin and some ciprofloxacin, but no high-speed antitoxins or vaccines. We are classified as a WMD-CST 'light,' meaning we are awaiting funding and training to be certified by the Department of Defense.

"That's the bad news."

The nervous captain paused.

"The good news is we are here and willing to help in any way possible. Our people are trained in biologic and chemical safety environments, and we have class A containment suits that we know how to use. Our medical non-commissioned officers are experienced field medics from the National Guard and the Air Guard, all with civilian health care experience as nurses or EMTs."

Captain Ledbetter continued.

"The strong point of our unit is our survey section, which has two teams of three soldiers trained to find the chemical and biologic sources that are plaguing the city, and control any booby-trap risks that might be associated with those sources.

"I'm sorry for the bad news part," he finished, "but please help direct us as to how we can help with the current situation with the tools that we do have."

Most of the crestfallen group numbly looked at the sincere young man who had entertained such high hopes for his unit before the dark cloud of botulism death had descended on Philadelphia.

Mateo grinned at the young Army captain.

"Our tests indicate the water supply is clean," Mateo said, "although the same cannot be said for the job of microwaving the diarrhea from the thousands of people in the Convention Center. As you might imagine, the detail is not a popular job among our young Marines. Captain Ledbetter, your men with class A suits will fit well into that task, and you may start your rotation at the next shift change."

"Yes, sir," agreed the young captain. "Consider it done."

Slidell was next to speak.

"We have asked for volunteers to work four-hour shifts providing assistance to the people in the Crisis Center, but we were disappointed to find only around two hundred willing people. When we broadcast that these volunteer health assistants would receive the Clostridium vaccine shot, the numbers quadrupled. The volunteers will begin to assist Dr. Mateo's team on the night shift tonight."

"Ms. Graves," Krause said, "how about the Red Cross?"

Melissa Graves stood.

"We have procured several thousand folding cots for the

Convention Center" she said, "and have good supplies of food for the patients and their family members. Our nurses have assisted with the Clostridium vaccine program, and more than ten thousand family members of the infected have received the immunization. Our supply and funding problems are minor compared to the hospital side of the incident."

She then sat quietly without mentioning that the communication area phone bill was already over $8,000 and that the food costs approached $10,000. She did not have the budget to support the added costs and hoped FEMA's pockets were deep enough to prevent her organization's embarrassment.

"Dr. Raines?" directed Krause.

Raines looked different. He was haggard, had two days growth of beard around his usually well-trimmed mustache, and was missing his usual grin and positive outlook. Ron Raines stood and delivered the devastating news.

"The epidemic of infectious botulism continues, though there are not as many deaths as in the first wave. We are treating the fluid loss and microwaving the infectious stool, but we have found that neither ciprofloxacin, ampicillin, nor sulfa drugs seem to slow the infection. Most of the antibiotic agents we've tried are nearly exhausted throughout the city, including the drugstores, as well as all the hospitals. It appears we may have to settle in for the long haul with this problem," he concluded.

The mood in the room was increasingly somber.

"Dr. Marshall?" called Krause as the meeting drew near its end.

Marshall slowly stood, scratched his dark, curly scalp and allowed the pause to prepare the group for the napalm blast of the Pennsylvania state lab's discovery.

"The agent responsible for the second wave of infection has been identified as an Enterobacter germ, a common gut microorganism that has been genetically given the power to produce pure botulinum toxin A," Marshall summarized.

"This can only mean one thing," he said. "This germ was engineered using advanced biotechnology— that is, gene-splicing techniques in which the genes for producing the toxin were added to a common gastrointestinal germ."

He automatically adjusted his glasses at every sentence.

"We will have to leave the police work of finding the production source to the Mr. Talbot and the police," he continued, "but it's clear that our only means of fighting this thing is to let the state laboratory help us find the antibiotics that will effectively kill this diabolically created germ. Until we get the results of the germ's sensitivities, we need to continue to isolate body fluids and prevent the germ's spreading from person to person in the population. My only remaining hope is that the lab in Pittsburgh will have tools for us to try once the final antibiotic sensitivities are available in a few days."

Chapter 37

DESPERATION

Philadelphia; 16–17 September 2008

When Ron Raines returned to Jefferson on the evening of September 16th, he fell straight into a chasm of frustration. The numbers of the botulism affected continued to swell, the buses to the Crisis Center continued to run, and the infection medication therapies he tried seemed to make little difference. The emergency re-supply from the naval hospitals and from Baxter Healthcare gave them intravenous fluids for more than twenty-four hours, but now even that supply was again running low.

I wonder if we should abandon the inner city and set up a new perimeter that might be free of the disease, he thought with desperation.

"Jorge! JORGE!" Raines heard a mother scream from the department's triage area. He rushed over, to see Christie beginning chest compressions on a young boy as Aphry from respiratory therapy used a mask and bag to ventilate the boy's thin body on the ER floor. Raines noted that the boy's too-large pants were held into place with a well-worn belt that was cinched tight to hold the garment in place. Raines knelt at the boy's head, took the laryngoscope and endotracheal tube offered by the respiratory therapist, and rapidly positioned the tube that provided the last shot at pushing oxygen into the patient's lungs. Raines then took over chest compressions as Christie struggled to establish an IV line in the thin boy's forearm.

Christie's experienced eyes searched the boy's skin for telltale traces of the underlying veins. She placed the small, 22-gauge catheter into an antecubital vein and saw the flash of blood in the needle hub that signaled successful access to the boy's circulatory system. She realized as she taped down the IV needle that she was thinking of Karen's daughters, so similar in age and almost as terribly affected by the monster microorganism.

Epinephrine, then atropine, then epinephrine again went through the tiny intravenous needle, and the boy's young and flexible chest wall was compressed to near its breaking point. The medications and breathing cycles repeated, but the monitor remained an unwavering flat line. The boy's heart failed to return to the propelling force that had enabled base-ball and street hockey.

After twenty minutes of attempting to change the flat lined EKG monitor," Raines said quietly to the mother, "I'm sorry, ma'am," "He's gone."

"He can't be gone!" the mother shrieked. "He is only eight years old!"

Raines turned from the impossible scene, seething with anger.

A paramedic lifted the young boy's body onto a transport gurney, and Raines watched as the boy and his oversized tennis shoes rolled into the distance.

It was just too much... This child was too much like the street kids, and Ron Raines knew that he was powerless to protect them. He wanted to be doing something important, but sometimes, trying to do the important still did not make a difference. Maybe this whole attempt was misguided, and they were truly beaten.

Christie looked into the face of the emergency physician and felt his distress.

"We can't quit, Ron!" she said quietly, placing her hand on his arm.

"... I know," he said finally.

She was right. The innocent depended on them to continue, to do their best to save lives with the limited tools they possessed. The street kids needed him to keep on keeping on.

⁓

At 8 p.m., Lawanda Burroughs was long past her usual bedtime. She had been reassigned to the Pennsylvania Crisis Center, and was lost in a sea of the critically ill. She understood living on strange hours, attending medical assistant classes at the Delaware Valley Academy each morning, sleeping during the afternoon, and working each night on the oncology ward of Pennsylvania University Hospital, but she had never been asked to do such tasks as breathe for another human being.

This day, and the stress that went with it, was taking its toll. She slowly compressed the Ambu bag in her hands, bringing air into the lungs of thirty-year-old Tom Savage, a maintenance worker for the City of Philadelphia. After nine hours, this new task had lost its foreign feel and had became a mind-numbing repetition. Breathe ... and watch as the pulses in Savage's neck continued their thump, thump, thump rhythm. Breathe ... thump, thump, thump. The heart plodded on if just given a little reason to keep trying.

Lawanda thought of her two young children at home and her own homework that was due on Friday.

Don't know if we'll have class, anyway. I guess it's okay to wait, she thought. Her head felt increasingly heavy, and she fought to keep her eyes focused on her task.

Lawanda Burroughs awoke with a start.

Did I fall asleep? her mind screamed. Breathe... no thump... Breathe... still no thump. In a panic, she felt for a pulse, and there was none. She opened the eyelids and looked into the unseeing pupils of Tom Savage.

"Nurse!" screamed Lawanda, "I can't feel a pulse!"

A nurse hurried over, though anxious to return to the more than one hundred patients already under her care. She felt the carotid artery for a pulse and then slowly shook her head.

"I'm sorry, hon," the nurse said, "but he's gone."

"He just can't be gone," Lawanda cried, "not like this!"

With a puzzled look, the nurse motioned for a Marine to move the body to the rear loading dock where the refrigeration truck and trailer awaited the dead.

Lawanda was distraught; she had failed in her first important task of caring for another human being. *"It's all my fault! I shouldn't even be here!"* thought Lawanda. *"I just need to go on back to my old job at the Circle K."*

"So now what?" she asked the nurse dejectedly.

The charge nurse took her by the shoulder and gave her a little hug.

"It's hard losing your first one, hon. Come on, this lady needs your help."

Lawanda went to sit in a chair beside the gurney of a fiftyish woman of matronly size, where she resumed the breathe... thump, thump, thump care that was now the most important thing on her earth.

～

At five p.m., Major Brad Tower entered the Pennsylvania Convention Center and as usual, stopped at the coffeepot in the Red Cross assistance area. Captain Mateo was always waiting for him here, but this evening was different. Although Tower waited until nearly six, his physician, mentor, and friend did not show. At five after six, Tower entered the sleeping area and headed for Mateo's bunk.

Tower saw the captain lying on his left side, one arthritic hand perched peacefully upon his chest, and his gray hairline unkempt over his old, weathered face.

"Hey, Skipper, time to rise and shine!" Tower began, and then noted, in horror, the gray discoloration of his adopted father's face. There was no reassuring, rhythmic movement of the chest, and the old man did not respond to his wake up call. Tower felt for a carotid pulse ... but the old sailor was already gone.

Chapter 38

BILAL CENTER

Houston, Texas; 17 September 2008

SAC Wells had been quite specific in his directions to the Houston team of FBI agents. The surveillance team's leader would be Special Agent Tommy Clinton, and they were to return to Philadelphia with suspects in custody.

"Get out to Texas," Wells directed. "Put the Islamic Center under surveillance, and find out how many accomplices we are dealing with and if they all remain in the area. You are not to intervene until we confirm the identities and are sure no one else is meeting them. We'll arrange search warrants while you're en route and arrest warrants once you get the names."

Special Agent Clinton sat quietly in coach class, weighing strategy for the arrest. Four gringo federal cops in suits would not be able to walk into the Bilal Center and demand infor-

mation on any Philadelphia-area terrorists who happened to
be visiting. There was no time to infiltrate an informant, thus
good old American greed would need to be the approach of
choice.

~

The FBI team landed at Houston's George Bush International and moved into surveillance mode. Agent Morris
stepped into the airport restroom and emerged in jeans,
T-shirt, and windbreaker, looking only a bit chubby due to the
Kevlar vest beneath the shirt. He purchased an orange Texas
Longhorns baseball cap at the airport gift shop to complete
his street appearance. The other agents remained in government approved suits and ties.

The four men picked up their rental car keys at the Hertz
counter and moved out to a gray Ford Mustang and a steel-
blue Range Rover waiting in the lot.

Special Agent Clinton drove the Mustang, with Morris as
his temporary passenger. Agent Ted Farmer piloted the Range
Rover and followed the Mustang at a respectable distance.
Agent Wall accompanied Farmer in the passenger seat. The
agents followed the Mapquest directions printout and arrived
at the Bilal Islamic Center of Houston just before one p.m.

Morris exited the Mustang a block before reaching the
center and ambled down the city streets, using a practiced eye
for hide locations, the Islamic Center vehicles, and the directions of all possible exits from the inner-city location.

Special Agents Farmer and Wall parked the Range Rover
in front of the Coventry Arms Apartments and Townhomes
building that stood on Waco Lane, across the street and facing
the side entrance of the Islamic Center. They entered the
business office, where they found a silver-haired Texas matri-
arch listening to country music radio and chain-smoking
Marlboros.

"Can I help you gents?" she drawled. It was not common to

see two dress-suited, muscular young men in the heart of an area that was less than the city's best neighborhood.

"We're looking for an apartment with a front view," Farmer asked politely. "Just for the month."

"I got four," the rough-hewn old Texan answered. "Take your pick."

She handed over four keys so that the men could select the apartment with the view that they preferred, which was the best covert view of the Islamic Center's side entrance.

As the men departed the office and climbed up the concrete stairs, the rental matron called to her husband in the living space behind the office.

"Hey, Earl," she drawled, "we already have to put up with the ragheads, and now the damn gays are takin over the neighborhood."

～

Special Agent Morris walked slowly around the corner in front of the Islamic Center and turned down Waco Lane, along the side of the Islamic Center. He observed the light brown Impala with the Avis rental sticker on the rear bumper parked near the doorway. He carefully noted its license plate and the newspapers on the car's rear shelf, indicating at least one person using the rear seat. He ambled to the end of the block and sat patiently on an empty city bus bench.

Clinton drove the Mustang through the area's adjacent blocks, noting each fast food restaurant, the video rental houses, and the convenience stores. He traced back the routes to the interstate exit and mapped out the fastest streets with the least traffic.

Agent Morris called Clinton's cell phone after spending only an hour on the bench.

"I have two males and a female exiting a van labeled Township Commercial Cleaning and entering the building through the Waco Lane entrance. Also at the site is an Avis rental, brown Chevrolet, license Texas CCK 458. No persons of interest visualized."

"I'm on it," noted Clinton, and hung up. He then called the Houston Police Department and asked for Lieutenant Scales.

"The FBI surveillance team is in position, and we appreciate your assistance," Clinton schmoozed. "We have a vehicle of interest and would appreciate the Avis rental information. The vehicle is a brown Chevrolet, Texas license CCK 458. I'd also appreciate the owner name and location for Township Commercial Cleaning."

"Will do," responded Scales as he checked his computer screen to locate the emergency contact for the cleaning business. "Township's owner is Charles Gray, and the office is at 409 Commerce Street, which is downtown off Broad Street. I'll run the car rental and call you back."

Clinton reversed the Mustang and headed for the downtown Houston business district. He had only traveled three blocks when he had another cell call from Morris.

"Four likely-looking males just exited the center's Waco Lane doorway and departed in the brown Chevrolet rental. They're headed west on Waco," Morris informed him.

Clinton pulled the Mustang into its second reversal and headed east on Waco Lane. Within five minutes, he spotted the Chevrolet as it pulled into a McDonald's that he had scouted just an hour earlier. Clinton circled the restaurant and parked the Mustang on the side opposite the rented Impala.

Clinton removed his tie, leaving on his suit coat to cover the FBI-issued Glock .40 caliber in the paddle holster on the belt behind his right hip. He entered the restaurant and stood in line to order, watching intently as the three young men took their food and chose a booth at the rear corner of the restaurant.

Clinton sat two tables away from the group and slowly dipped fries in ketchup. He noted that a bearded man, who frequently looked about as if for security risks, seemed to do most of the talking. A second bearded man had apparently suffered a severe burn, leaving him only one eye and a disfigured face. The youngest man sported a moustache. Clinton was able to make out the name "Farouk" from the speech of the leader to the younger man. He understood little else, for the entire conversation was in Arabic. As Clinton ate quietly and watched, his cell phone chirped.

"Hello," Clinton answered simply, surprising Lieutenant Scales by avoiding his usual clipped greeting of "Clinton."

"The brown Chevrolet was rented in Texas City, Texas on September 12 by a Ahmed Madawi of Apartment 11D, 467 Waycross, Philadelphia." Scales gave Agent Clinton the MasterCard number that was used for the rental, and read off the registration of the card: "Delaware Bay Benevolence Fund. Is that helpful?"

"You betcha," responded Clinton as he finished scribbling down the information on a napkin. "Gotta run. Thanks."

The three Middle Eastern men were already exiting their table, not bothering to stow the trash from the meal in the nearby can. They wordlessly walked to the parking lot, got into the Impala, and turned to the east on Waco.

"They're moving," Clinton hit the speed dial on his cell phone and said to Morris. "You've got the ball."

Special Agent Clinton called the Philadelphia FBI's operations center as he drove to the Township Commercial Cleaning Company.

"We need a make on an Al-Douri member with the name 'Farouk'," he requested. He passed along the name Ahmed Madawi and the Benevolence Fund MasterCard number and requested that a team of agents search for the attack truck in the used-vehicle lots in Texas City, Texas.

"We have three likelys thus far: two bearded and in their thirties, one early twenties and clean-shaven. One of the older men has distinguishing scars and one eye. We're attempting an inside contact through a cleaning service and have the Islamic Center under surveillance from an apartment across the street, plus a 'walker' in the neighborhood. I'll forward my written report by secure e-mail tonight."

~

Around four, Clinton arrived at the Township Commercial Cleaning office, presented his credentials, and asked to see Mr. Gray. He was ushered into a squalid office that reeked of cigars, inhabited by a large man in his sixties with a handlebar moustache and a "Don't Mess with Texas" belt buckle. The man appeared puzzled but unafraid as Clinton presented his credentials and proceeded directly to the discussion.

"We have an establishment under observation, and your cleaning service was there today," Clinton began. "We have interest in some of the individuals who may be living at this location and can offer a reward for the names of these individuals and where in the building they can be found."

"What is the establishment?" asked Gray.

"The Bilal Islamic Center."

"Hell, I should've known those people were up to no good," Gray responded. "My cleaning crew will be back here in a couple of hours, and I'll arrange for Alice to get your information. She could use the money, anyway. Hell, I'm a Vietnam vet, and I don't want no damn foreigners messing with things I went to Southeast Asia for."

Chapter 39

RENDITION

Incirclik, Turkey; 17 September 2008

The op is a go," repeated Deputy Director Green via the encrypted satellite link to the handset held by Stroud on the Gulfstream. The CIA Director and White House nod occurred on September 17 at nine a.m., and an hour later, the deputy director "passed the team the ball."

It was five p.m. on the 17th in Turkey, but Zulu time would be in effect for the duration of the mission, and the go/no-go decision in eight hours. In addition to Stroud, Thomas, Becker, and Lopez were already up. The Geek was stretched out in his plush aircraft seat; glasses carefully perched on his chest.

Wills stretched across the aisle and gave the Geek a rousing kick in the calf.

"Get up, Sleeping Beauty," he prodded with brotherly concern.

"Thirty minutes till wheels up, gentlemen—and sunup is in eleven and a half hours," directed Stroud as he walked to the aft area of the cabin that housed his team. "We go weapons red only upon landing at the destination."

The team moved into high gear, stuffing final MRE's—or "Meals Rejected by Everyone—and ammunition into the camping backpacks that were already prepared for the Russian helicopter. The Geek made a final battery check and then put his satellite-linked BGAN laptop into its padded leather case. He then passed off an iridium hand-held satellite phone to the colonel to retain communication with Washington should he or the laptop be killed or captured.

Becker packed his six half-kilogram timer charges as Lopez readied his medical kit, including the injectable lorazepam calculated for Atoomb's estimated body weight. Lopez would "sleep" him only if he were uncooperative.

Thomas lovingly zipped the case on his M-14 and placed a strong brown arm through the special strap that suspended the weapon behind his right shoulder like a natural extension of his body.

Wills grinned like a schoolboy seeing his first breast.

"Remember, this is a rendition, and we *must* have him alive," Stroud reminded as he looked directly at the young "Swabbie."

"Shoot, Colonel," grinned Wills, "you know I'm a pacifist at heart."

The Special Activities Team walked down the boarding ramp of the Gulfstream, moving rapidly despite their individual loads of backpacks and weapons. Turkey in September was cold during the early evening hours, and the ski parkas and padded ski pants provided not only warmth but also cover and concealment for side arms and lightweight Kevlar vests. Per the commander's instruction, the group confirmed empty weapon chambers as they left the aircraft.

The HIP Mi-17 helicopter's main rotor blades thumped in the still-dark Turkish air. Its pitch was lower and throatier than an American Chinook or Blackhawk helicopter due to its pair of 1900-horsepower Isotov turboshaft engines. The craft was still Russian-issue camouflage and had required little modification for its CIA service. It came from the Russian factory equipped with Doppler radar useful for the Caspian coast weather and featured electronic warfare countermeasures, including chaf and flare pods. The Russian PUS-31-71 fire control system had been modified to control the American HELLFIRE missiles and the pair of American M61A1 Vulcan 20mm mini-guns. The Vulcan's impressive 6,000-round-per-minute firepower made only a ripping sound when fired, as the rotating barrels of the Gatling gun sent rounds downrange too rapidly to break down into their individual "pops." The eight AGM-114C HELLFIRE missiles could wreak havoc from four miles away, hitting the target without fail due to their "Lock before Launch" laser guidance. The target could be "lazed" by a beam from the helicopter's pilot or by the ten-inch, hand-held PEQ-4 laser illuminators that both Stroud and Becker carried.

The plan, however, did not call for the use of all this firepower. The craft would slip in at twenty feet above the Caspian Sea and at almost 150 miles per hour, and would then make two false insertions before landing in the Chalus River Gorge. Stealth was the primary tool and the Agency's pilots had learned it from the best. All of the Special Activities Division's rotary wing aviators were graduates of the U.S. Army's 160th Special Operations Aviation Regiment—elite "Night Stalkers." Almost all of each pilot's flying for the 160th was at NOE, nape of the earth levels, and under night vision goggles. By 160th convention, the pilots never used a last name or rank, just their first-name designation chosen for the mission and only given to the team commander. The Mi-17's pilot for this event simply called himself "Frank."

The six team members entered the rear clamshell doors and spread out, three to each aircraft side. The center of the cargo area held two strapped-down Iranian 125cc Scig motorcycles, fitted with snow tires and heavy-duty batteries. The craft lifted its relatively light load quickly and was soon wheels up and disappearing into the dark Eastern sky.

As the helicopter rocketed toward its Ali Bayramli, Azerbaijan refueling, Stroud put on the intercom headset, thanked the pilot for his time and expertise, and confirmed the GPS coordinates of the refueling and landing sites. The Geek opened his laptop, rapidly made the satellite uplink, and tapped out a single-word, encrypted e-mail to the Special Activities Division in Washington.

The message read: "Inbound."

~

At 10:20 p.m. Azerbaijani time, the craft circled the refueling coordinates, and the pilot saw the flashing of four infrared strobes switched on at the corners of a paved, rectangular landing pad. As the Russian craft's wheels settled onto the pad, only Stroud moved to the exit and disembarked into the night.

"Evenin," drawled the voice of a Texas oilman through the cold East Asia darkness. "You boys need some gas?"

"We'd be very appreciative," responded Stroud, without unnecessary introductions or discussion of his destination.

The oilman slid the nozzle of the JP-8 fuel line into the helicopter without even having to ask for the location of the extended-range tanks. A second man exited a tin building just visible in the dark and extended to Stroud a pair of thermoses filled with hot Texas coffee.

"Y'all kick some ass, now, y'hear," said the second man as he disappeared into the refueling shanty.

Stroud smiled and reentered the aircraft with a wave of

thanks to the pump man, his heart strangely warmed by a piece of America residing in such an alien place.

After the two-hour, course altering run across the oil spill and DDT-polluted Caspian, the Mi-17 crossed the border into Iran. The craft turned south for two false insertions before passing into the River Gorge at 00:10 a.m. local time. Frank piloted the craft down the gorge at nine feet above the ground and then landed and ground-taxied the craft beneath a copse of overhanging trees.

"This okay, Charlie?" he asked before shutting down the twin turbo-shaft engines.

Stroud double-checked his hand-held GPS and gave Frank the thumbs up for the shutdown. The sun's rise over the Caspian was five hours away.

"We depart the aircraft at 0030 hours and pick up the van twenty minutes later," said Stroud simply. "You may go weapons hot and make your final checks." In twenty minutes, Stroud would make the 2200 Zulu encrypted satellite call to Washington using a "burst" transmission that lasted less than one-half of a second. The operation would be approved.

Chapter 40

CUFFS

Texas and Pennsylvania; 18 September 2008

At 8:20 a.m. in Houston, Texas, a chime sounded, alerting Clinton to the receipt of a secure e-mail message. He opened the file to view the arrest warrant for one Ahmed Madawi of South Philadelphia, plus Mohammed and Farouk Rahman of Camden, New Jersey. Clinton printed the document and carefully laid it on top of the search warrant that awaited service.

"Lieutenant Scales, please," Clinton spoke into his cell phone as his fellow agents buckled on Kevlar in preparation for the raid.

"Three suspects are in the center and we hold a warrant," Clinton reported. "Let's move in at 1000 hours."

Next, he called Morris, who was still sitting on his now familiar bus bench on the corner of Waco Lane.

"We go at ten. Warrant is on hand for three, plus the search of the center. Local backup has been arranged."

Morris reported his readiness and double-checked his watch.

At 09:59 a.m., six Houston police cruisers raced into the parking lot of the Bilal Islamic Center with lights flashing, but eerie silence underscoring the absence of sirens. The four FBI agents entered the center, presenting credentials as they walked rapidly past a shocked young clerk sitting at a reception desk, and continued directly to the dormitory room. Only Mohammed was awake as the four armed men in FBI Kevlar burst through the door of the room.

Mohammed, seated at a small desk, was reading the Haditha as the threat entered. He reached beneath the desk for the loaded Makarov but never got the chance to fire it. The last thing he saw was a man in a Texas Longhorn baseball cap leveling a .40 caliber Glock at his face. Less than a second later, that man placed a round through Mohammed's forehead and two through his heart.

The groggy Faithful, awakened by their brother's sudden demise, sat with open mouths but no threatening movements. The two remaining Faithful were handcuffed, and still in shock, led to the waiting police cruisers.

~

Special Agent Deason used an advanced FBI investigative technique in Texas City, Texas: he bought a newspaper. In the "Used Trucks and Vans" section of the paper's classified ads was an advertisement for a 1994 International truck with 230,000 miles that "needs work but runs good."

Deason's partner, Agent Semmes, revived his old cowboy hat and purchased a tin of Skoal to assist with the investigation. In jeans and a T-shirt, he entered the Paris Wrecking Yard to inquire about the truck for sale.

Hollis Rampart looked over his potential customer, doubtful

that the man could come up with the $12,000 price, and silently rose from his cluttered desk.

"The truck's out back," he offered. "Don't really want to sell it, but things have been a mite tough in the dredging business lately."

"How does it run?" asked Semmes a moment later as he climbed into the cab and confirmed the vehicle identification number mounted on the dashboard. He deftly swiped a SMART ticket across the brake and clutch pedals as he pretended to check their wear and action.

"It runs good for an older model," reported Rampart truthfully.

Semmes circled around to the back of the truck and called, "Hey, do you mind tripping the turn signals and brake lights while I check in back?"

Rampart grudgingly climbed into the cab. He pumped the brakes and clicked each turn signal as Semmes rubbed down the rear bumper and rear trailer lip with a fresh SMART ticket.

"That looks good," called Semmes. "Why don't you start 'er up?"

The old diesel cranked on the first try, but Semmes really didn't see the need to take it around the block. He didn't plan to buy; he planned to get an arrest warrant.

～

Imam Derwish's eyes opened wide when he heard the words that came from Special Agent Landrum's mouth.

"Arrest? On what charge?" Derwish stammered.

"Conspiracy, money laundering, and accessory to murder," listed Landrum as he placed the cuffs on the holy man's wrists.

"This is an insult to Islam!" yelled the imam.

"This has nothing to do with Islam," replied Special Agent Landrum. "This concerns terrorist activities that cost the lives of more than two thousand Philadelphia citizens."

Chapter 41

ROUND UP

Texas and Arkansas; 18 September 2008

Hollis Rampart stood on the deck of his rusting work barge, watching with trepidation as three dress-suited men crossed the gangway and approached his partly finished welding. These men dressed too well to be customers of the Paris Dredging Company, leaving only the business with the Arabs and his occasional smuggling of marijuana as possible topics for any discussions with the "suits."

"Hollis Rampart," said Special Agent Tony Semmes, showing credentials and removing all questions of his real interest in the truck. "FBI," he said bluntly. "You are under arrest for the possession of a vehicle used in a felony, plus accessory to murder."

"Oh hell," Rampart, "that sounds *real* serious."

Over the next hour, Hollis Rampart handed over the keys

to the International truck that remained parked in its original spot near the rear of the dredging company. He helpfully showed the agents the marine chart that pinpointed the offshore location of his dumpsite, and described the container and the body that the Arabs had tried to hide from him. He volunteered to testify as a state's witness against the Arabs in exchange for later consideration in his own hearing.

$\sim$

In Pine Bluff, Arkansas, the street address of the Biolimit Corporation was an abandoned old house adjacent to an aging grain elevator. A neighbor down the street told the FBI agents that the adult children of an elderly man who died six or eight years before had abandoned the house.

Special Agent Deason checked the Pine Bluff post office records for the phone number of the person or persons who rented the Biolimit mailbox, but none was available. His only approach was to wait patiently for someone to pick up the mail.

After two days of sitting inside the post office watching the backside of a mailbox, he was rewarded with the clicking of the box combination. Agent Deason then watched from the inside as the mailbox door opened to reveal a portion of the face of a young woman with her head covered by a silk scarf.

Deason moved through the post office's door into the customer lobby, intercepting the woman who was departing with mail in hand.

"FBI," stated Deason, flashing his credentials. "You are to accompany me to the Pine Bluff police headquarters for questioning. Are you alone?"

"No ... ah ..." she answered, with a revealing glance toward an old pickup in the parking lot that contained a skinny Asian male and two small children.

Deason nodded to the agent assisting him, who called in a backup request to the Pine Bluff police and then stepped into the parking lot with weapon drawn to apprehend the driver of the truck.

~

In the Pine Bluff police station, Deason held the young Filipino Muslims in separate interrogation rooms. He held his first conversation with Mrs. Pitong.

"Your mail today contains your personal bills and local advertisements," he began, "but your mailbox is also listed as the mailing address of the Biolimit Corporation. What is your connection to Biolimit, and why do you share a mailbox with that company?"

"I've never heard of this company," she answered truth-fully, revealing that her husband rented the mailbox and that she had been to the post office only on a few occasions. After an hour, Deason was convinced that the frightened young mother had no knowledge of a vaccine company residing in her mailbox.

"I know of this Biolimit," Mr. Pitong confided during his own interrogation, "only because I was paid to mail letters for them. The letters were typed, sealed, and stamped when they were delivered to me."

"How many letters?" demanded Deason.

"Three or four," offered Pitong. "I was given twenty dollars each to mail them."

"Why would someone pay you more than the cost of the box rent just to *mail* a letter and *receive* mail for a company, rather than just get a box for himself?" yelled Deason.

"I do not know, Officer," replied the shaking Filipino, "but it is true!"

"Who gave you the letters?" Deason demanded.

"A friend at the mosque, Mr. Ahmadi," replied Pitong. "He runs a dry-cleaning business on Yong Street."

"I have no further questions for you today," Deason concluded. "You are free to go but are forbidden to leave the city, in case you are needed for additional questioning."

After the nearly innocent young couple left, Deason checked the records of Pine Bluff business owners. He then placed a call to Special Agent Landrum in Philadelphia.

"I need a Warrant ASAP," requested Deason, "for a Leonard Ahmadi, 239 Yong Street, Pine Bluff, Arkansas. The charge is international transport of a deadly weapon and accessory to murder."

Chapter 42

THE SNATCH

Tehran, Iran; 18 September 2008

At 0030 hours local time, in the Chalus River Gorge of the Iranian Elburz Mountains, the Special Activities Team quietly went about final preparations for the mission. There were no alarms or orders needed, and the highly professional group of men simply moved into their own mental game plans when the time came. Weapons remained in backpacks, and side arms underwent a final check. The motorcycles were unstrapped and rolled out the clamshell doors of the Mi-17 into the cold mountain air.

At 0030 hours, the team was ready and waiting. Stroud looked around the aircraft and gave each man the opportunity for final questions or comments.

"Let's do it," announced Stroud, and the team exited the aircraft.

Bearded Becker and mustachioed Lopez mounted the bikes, each riding solo for the entirety of the trip into Tehran. The team rapidly covered the six miles to the ancient orange-and-white van, hidden at the arranged GPS location in the high grass and trees off one of the hunting trails that wound through the gorge. The van started easily, and Stroud and the Geek climbed into the rear seat. Wills drove the frighteningly old, but situation appropriate van, with Thomas and his precious M-14 riding shotgun. At 0055 hours, the van and its accompanying pair of motorcycles reentered the trail and headed northwest toward Tehran.

The streets were nearly deserted as they entered the city of nine million, for morning prayers were still five hours away. Only five hours left to remove one citizen from his morning plans for the prayer rug.

As they entered the city, a few lights blazed in late-night shops, and an occasional orange-and-white taxi passed them at breakneck speed. Lopez's motorcycle pulled ahead, remaining within sight of the van, as Becker dropped back to provide rear guard support. The convoy wound through the narrow streets, through discarded plastic bags, cardboard boxes and past flowing streams of sewage, until they reached the Marzook Apartments building.

The van backed into the driveway as though making a delivery, and Wills left the engine running. The four team members from the van pulled on fiberglass assault helmets with mounted night-vision devices and rapidly moved into the shadows of the building.

Becker circled the building on the small bike, dismounted, and stationed himself beneath Atoomb's apartment window. The window hovered more than thirty feet above the sidewalk, but a jump was not out the question for a desperate man. Becker placed two of his mini-charges along the rear of the building to act as a diversion if the team were compromised.

The team ran across the first-floor courtyard to the stairwell leading to the second floor. The Geek remained near the entrance to the stairs with eyes on the van, as Stroud and the remaining four team members rapidly passed him and climbed to the second floor.

Lopez took his position crouched by Atoomb's door as Wills dropped to one knee and began to pick the door's lock and the deadbolt above. Thomas provided cover as he crouched with his deadly M-14 behind the railing of the landing, peering with expert eyes into the quiet courtyard of the apartment building.

In less than two minutes, the door swung open, and Stroud and Wills dashed inside, followed by Thomas. The soft glow of a bathroom light made the night-vision devices glow uncomfortably bright, and Thomas snapped the light off, as would a father preparing his family for bed. Stroud and Wills quietly entered the only bedroom, flanked by Thomas, and found Atoomb still asleep.

Stroud reached down and grabbed a handful of the scientist's hair, jerking Atoomb to his feet. The man's eyes flew open to see the dull green glow of the night-vision devices over the eyes of three very serious men, one of whom pointed directly at his chest a weapon that looked as large as cannon. Stroud noticed the stain of warm urine appearing on the baggy pants covering Atoomb's shaking legs.

"You are under arrest for the murder of more than two thousand citizens of Philadelphia, Pennsylvania," said Stroud quietly in English, "and the attempted murder of an additional two thousand. If you make one sound or attempt to resist, I promise that I will not kill you; I will blow off your balls one at a time."

Wills rapidly placed plastic FlexiCuffs over the scientist's wrists and pulled them tight. He then placed a thin nylon hood over Atoomb's head and secured it with a band of duct tape over the mouth and behind the neck.

Wills roughly grabbed the FlexiCuffed wrists and leaned

in near the hooded head.

"I don't promise you any damn thing," he hissed, and pulled Atoomb to the apartment door.

Stroud and Wills pulled Atoomb rapidly down the stairs, collecting Lopez as they exited. Thomas remained on his perch of death until the group had removed helmets and night devices and stowed Atoomb on the rear floor of the van. The aging rifleman then rapidly moved down the stairs and took his shotgun position in the van. The vehicle exited the apartment complex eight minutes after its arrival.

Becker remounted his Scig and followed the van, leaving the charges on the rear of the apartment building. If someone attacked the convoy, he could still radio-detonate the diversion from up to three miles away. Lopez passed the van on his motorcycle, and the group moved cautiously through the dirty, winding streets toward eastern Tehran.

~

Ali Quatami sat in his video shop in east Tehran during the early morning hours. The hour made little difference, since he had few customers at three a.m., and just as few during daylight hours. Selling copied videos had never been much of a source of money, perhaps because of the economy, perhaps because of the quality of his wares. He sent the street boys into the American and Japanese movies playing in Tehran to make copies of the films with a cheap, handheld video camera. The films were grainy and clearly were taken inside a theater; they included the sounds of crying children and viewers' coughs. The sound was a bit tinny and frequently lost quality in the mass recopy procedure. Only the labels for the cheap DVD cases were of good quality, since they were pirated from the Internet photos advertising the movie.

These financial realities were the reason Quatami supplemented his business income by being a police informant. He shared information on his neighbors and customers and then watched them being carted off, never to be heard from again. He knew there was a payment possible in the convoy he now saw crawling through the darkened, early morning streets of Tehran.

"Lieutenant Bushehr, please," Quatami requested politely, and then he waited patiently for the local Iranian Imperial Police officer.

"Yes?" answered Bushehr, smirking at the lack of ethics that enabled Quatami to inform on his neighbors.

"Lieutenant, I have valuable information on an illegal group of vehicles headed east on Harrakat Street," reported the businessman. "The vehicle is an orange-and-white taxi van and carries four men, with the driver a red-headed man who looks like an infidel American. Motorcycles both lead and follow the van for protection. They headed west on Harrakat twenty minutes ago and now are returning to the east."

"And who are these criminals, Quatami?" asked the cautious policeman.

"That I do not know, Lieutenant," Quatami admitted, "but I am sure that they must be enemies of the Republic!"

"I will be in touch … if your information has value," ended Bushehr. He turned to his junior officer and ordered the preparation of a truck and police squad.

The five Iranian Imperial Police soldiers, armed with AK-47's and Zoaf 9mm pistols, climbed into the back of the worn Mercedes truck as Bushehr climbed in beside the driver.

"East on Harrakat, quickly," directed the middle-aged lieutenant.

The aging truck coughed and clattered into eastern Tehran.

"We have company, Charlie," noted Wills as he watched the truck's headlights first light up Becker, then the rear of the van.

"Maintain your current speed," directed Stroud, "and we'll

pull them into a place of our choosing."

The rendition convoy continued its passage through the eastern city and entered the agricultural land on the city's fringe. Stroud picked up the Iridium phone and dialed Frank's number.

"Single vehicle tail," he related. "Mercedes truck with armed men in the rear, current location 32-48 North, 53-69 West. Final coordinates to follow."

Frank started the Mi-17 engines during the last seconds of Stroud's call.

"ETA six minutes," reported Frank with his usual professionalism. The camouflaged helicopter ground-taxied from beneath its tree-covered hide site and took off to the west while still rolling forward. Frank kept the craft at a 150-foot elevation as the helicopter's nose dipped and the airspeed indicator climbed to 140 miles per hour. Within four minutes, the lights of eastern Tehran grew near.

"How about that spot?" suggested Thomas, pointing to a barley field off the right front of the van.

Stroud noted the absence of overhanging power lines, the slight rise to the land near the rear of the field, and the dusty entrance road guarded by a single strand of sagging barbed wire.

"Yeah, that looks good," agreed Stroud.

Wills jerked the wheel to the right, and the van slammed through the wire and into the open field. As Stroud updated Frank on their final GPS coordinates, Wills drove the van cross-country to the rear of the field, skidding to a halt on the small rise. Lopez and Thomas exited the vehicle, followed by Stroud, who slapped an infrared beacon to the top of the van to assure their visibility to the incoming visitor.

Wills remained at the wheel with the van's engine running, while the Geek pointed his MP-5 out the van's rear window and kept his right foot planted squarely on Atoomb's back, pressing him even more uncomfortably into the floor. Thomas positioned the M-14 across the short hood of the van as Stroud leveled his MP-5 from the rear of the vehicle.

"Ah, perhaps they do have things to hide," smiled Bushehr as the truck bounced across the rows of late fall barley. "Close enough," he waved to the driver, and the truck stopped eighty meters from the idling van.

"With haste!" he yelled to the soldiers in the truck. They scrambled out and dropped onto the dusty field.

"You three, to the right ..." he shouted, but the throaty rumble of a monster winging in from the eastern sky drowned out his orders. Like a prehistoric bird of prey, the chopper remained deceptively quiet until the time arrived for release of its fury.

The Mi-17 slowed to eighty miles per hour as it reached a quarter-mile distance from the field. The pilot's night-vision helmet gave a daylight-green glow to the truck with its offloading troops and a brilliant green blaze to the infrared strobe atop the van. As Frank lined up for the attack run, a thin laser line shot from Stroud at the rear of the van and centered on the hood of the Mercedes truck. The pilot locked the HELLFIRE missile onto the designator's infrared frequency and fired a single, seven-inch-diameter nightmare.

The missile slammed into the front of the Mercedes truck, exploding it into in a fireball that threw the truck's bed more than fifty meters toward the entrance to the barley field. The Mi-17 slowly passed over the burning wreckage and banked left, as Frank switched the fire control computer to the Vulcan for the gun run.

The pilot's helmet-mounted night device focused on the four men who were still attempting to crawl away from the burning hell on earth. The multi-barreled mini-gun tracked the movement of his helmet and placed the crawlers directly in the line of fire. As the craft lazily looped back into the filed, Frank fired a six-second burst, sending more than five thousand rounds the size of kindergarten pencils slamming into the earth and the men who were trying to escape. The night-vision device registered smoking heaps of bright green where crawling men had been a few seconds before.

The Mi-17 made a final pass with no further movement from the area where the truck had once been parked. Frank settled the chopper onto its wheels between the van and the field's entrance road.

Becker and Lopez then entered the field on their bikes and raced across the dusty barley as Frank opened the rear doors of the craft. Both bikes raced up the ramp, skidded to a halt, and then shut down in the cargo area

Stroud was the next to reach the Mi-17's rear doors, followed by Thomas and Wills at a run, dragging a still quaking Atoomb between them. The burly pair pulled Atoomb up the ramp, and Stroud, followed by the Geek, climbed aboard. Stroud hit the hydraulic lift to raise the ramp and close the clamshell doors, then gave Frank the thumbs-up for takeoff.

"Nothing like a rescue by the cavalry," Stroud shouted into the headset.

"All in a night's work, Colonel," replied the pilot.

The craft rocketed to the northeast at more than 150 miles per hour. In less than ten minutes, they were twelve miles out into the Caspian Sea at a flight altitude of thirty feet—and headed home.

Chapter 43

POTUS

The Oval Office revealed much of the personality of President Jack Lunsford; it spoke of power and professionalism. The office rug was a bold blue, with the Presidential Seal surrounded by beige-and-gold sunburst décor left over from the George W. Bush administration. The walls spoke of history and purpose, with a portrait of President George Washington over the fireplace mantle and the portrait of Abraham Lincoln to the right of the historic *HMS Resolute* desk. Smaller paintings of Harrier jump jets and the Mekong River completed the visitor's background on the things reflecting that this leader was decisive and in control.

President Lunsford was young—fifty-eight—and firmly believed that "there are no former Marines." He had been a Marine pilot and he always would be; and he ran the presidential office with a leatherneck's expectations for service and sacrifice.

As the afternoon sun began to slant across the Oval Office wall, the president looked up as his chief of staff entered.

"Kent, set up the Iranian ambassador for nine tomorrow morning," the president said. "I need to see the French and Norwegian ambassadors to follow—and we won't be serving breakfast to any of the bastards."

"Done, Mr. President," the trusted aide responded. "The press is ready in the Rose Garden, and Judge Aquino is here."

The president rose from the desk and followed the staff boss into the Executive Branch hallway.

～

"...and I challenge you to avoid petty party bickering in the confirmation hearings and to confirm this fine jurist's presence on our nation's highest court," President Lunsford concluded.

There was polite applause for the beaming Judge Aquino, who received the usual presidential slap on the back and departed the podium.

"Mr. President ..." began the chaos of voices in near unison. The president pointed to an old friend from the Associated Press.

"Is it true that there is evidence of Iranian involvement in the recent attack on the city of Philadelphia?"

"At this point," said President Lunsford, "we see clear links to support or simple tolerance in several European and Middle Eastern governments. The perpetrators of this criminal activity may have been acting in accordance with political or religious beliefs, however, the United States considers the attack an unprovoked act of war and will follow the necessary steps for our protection."

"Mr. President," asked a reporter from CNN, "what is the

expected death toll from the attack?"

"The current losses total more than two thousand lives, and there are thousands who remain critically ill," responded the president. "Obviously, we have no crystal ball for predicting the future numbers of our countrymen dying, but we have all federal, state, military, and civilian resources at work to save the citizens of Philadelphia. We are also taking steps to isolate the city and prevent the spread of the infection to other areas of the northeast."

"Mr. President," a man from *USA Today* asked, "Are you aware of the specific groups of terrorists that may be behind this attack?"

"Yes" was the simple answer from a straightforward leader.

"And who are those groups?" questioned the *Washington Post*.

"You will be introduced to them at their trials," responded the president with finality.

Chapter 44

INTERROGATION

Over Turkey, 18 September 2008

Winging over Turkey at six hundred miles per hour in the Gulfstream, the Special Activities Team enjoyed the deeply cushioned luxury of the jet. Their new cargo was not nearly as comfortable, with hands cuffed to his seat's arms and his feet cuffed together. Stroud nodded to Wills, who stood threateningly close to Dr. Khalid Atoomb.

Wills slipped a lightweight, folding combat knife from his right rear pocket, and with a deft flick of the right thumb snapped the locking, six-inch blade into an open position. The highly polished, razor-like surface of the knife reflected the cabin lights directly into Atoomb's eyes.

"We didn't come all the way to Iran just to toss you out of this plane for refusing to tell us what we need to know," said Wills flatly. "But I know from previous experience that you will still be able to speak just fine without your testicles."

Atoomb considered the actions already carried out by the team and felt that the promise was believable. He started at the beginning and told the "Jihad Germ" story in its entirety.

After two hours, Stroud picked up the receiver of a secure satellite phone in the sleeping cabin.

"He's singing like a bird," he related to Deputy Director Green. "The organism was produced over a two-year period with the assistance of expatriate Soviet biowarfare scientists in a facility buried deep beneath the Fathu al-Shamal fertilizer factory in Tehran. The bacterial stock of toxin-producing Clostridium was obtained from the American Type Culture Collection via an Arkansas shell company called Biolimit, reportedly for research into vaccine production.

"After their production, the toxin and recombinant germs were put into the false floor of a new shipping container," reported Stroud. "The shipment moved by rail to Bandar e-Abbas and into the port of Shahid Fajai. An Islamic Republic freighter transported it to Marseilles, where it was labeled with the packaging materials of a French shell company called Logis Sourient. The two thousand liters of recombinant germs and botulinum toxin then entered the United States in early September onboard the *Sonjnafiorden*, a Norwegian container ship, and entered the United States through the Port of Philadelphia. I think you are well aware of the rest of the story in Pennsylvania."

"So who's behind this?" demanded Green.

"Atoomb fingers an Iranian Intelligence general named Madmudiyeh as his immediate supervisor and reports personal contact with the Iranian Committee of Counselors. The links to the government are crystal clear and will be easy to prove."

"How about the Brotherhood of Islamic Jihad, the Muslim Benevolence Fund, and the Muslim Liberation Front?" asked Green.

"Atoomb has little if any knowledge of the financing of the operation or the source of orders for the attack. I'm convinced he is not aware, sir," Stroud advised.

"By the way, Mr. Director," he concluded, "tell the docs in Philadelphia that they can kill this germ with something called imipenem."

The director asked for the spelling of the drug's name and wrote it on his yellow legal pad.

"Good job, Charlie," smiled Green. "The lone survivor of the barley field event is reporting that they were lured into a trap by spies and then attacked by the Soviets. I see no reason to correct him. We will take custody of Dr. Atoomb at Camp Peary around 1800 hours Eastern Time. Travel safely."

Charlie Stroud hung up the secure line and mentally replayed the operation. They must have been spotted entering the city, and the motorcycle entourage may have contributed. However, no shots were fired near civilians, and the team was safe. The cargo was providing valuable information. Overall, he could consider the operation a success, but why didn't he feel good about it?

Only a sociopath could end the lives of other men without a second thought mused Stroud. It was an undeniable truth that those men were scared and desperately trying to crawl away. These men had mothers, probably had children, and would not be coming home. It might have been morally appropriate to leave them in the land of the living, but that risked the team's extraction. It also risked the "cargo" who could save lives in the United States. It was unavoidable evil: the decision to kill for the greater good. He guessed the view of what constituted the greater good was different on the other end of a HELLFIRE missile.

Chapter 45

IMIPENEM

Philadelphia; 19 September 2008

The night seemed unending. The botulism cases continued to stream in during the early-morning hours of September 18. Fever, diarrhea, and weakness were universal, though fewer people required assistance in breathing. An additional 240 people needed the care of the crisis center, and some of them would die, particularly since the center had again exhausted its supply of the antitoxin that had enabled many of the earliest cases to be weaned from respiratory assistance.

Raines felt hopeless. The therapies were ineffective; the population near panic, and no relief was in sight. When the hour was at its darkest, Raines heard a call—"Hey … Doc!"—from a hallway near triage.

In the darkened doorway stood Talbot, still in a wrinkled suit, despite the fact that it was almost two in the morning.

"Got some info that might be useful," offered the agency man. "You got a quiet place to talk?"

"This way," answered Raines. He led the way to the emergency department call room. The room was empty, but Raines noted Talbert's long-practiced visual scan for security and his mental acceptance of the accommodations.

"The most useful drug for this infection is ..." Talbot referred to his scribbles in a small, spiral-bound notebook "... something called ... imipenem."

"Imipenem?" exclaimed Raines. "How did you get the drug sensitivities before the lab even called Marshall?"

"My sources are outside of the laboratory, doc," grinned Talbot, planning to provide no more information than necessary.

Raines saw the hesitation on Talbot's face and added, "I still hold an army top-secret security clearance, you know."

Talbot shrugged and then offered some information.

"A scientist who was involved with the recombination technology creating this germ has fallen into the hands of my colleagues. He seems quite anxious to cooperate with information."

Although he had more questions, Raines sensed that Talbot would balk at providing anything further.

"Thanks a lot, Agent Talbot," he said genuinely. "I'll put your information to use right now."

~

"Well, looks like we have forty-one gram doses in house," reported Jefferson University Hospital's night pharmacist. "We could stretch it to eighty by using a more moderate 500 milligram dose."

"Thanks," sighed Raines. "Let's mix them all at the 500-milligram dose. Could you check with the other guys in town who might stock the drug?"

"Will do," the pharmacist replied, "and I'll have the

imipenem up to the ER in less than an hour."

The drug arrived as promised, and Raines dosed all of the forty-four botulism cases still in the ER.

"I've carefully marked the charts of those who received the new drug," he said to Christie, "and I'll call Marshall and let them know they should be watched in a separate area of the Crisis Center."

~

Marshall sat on the side of the bed in the makeshift sleeping area to the rear of the Convention Center.

"Imipenem!" said Marshall, smiling. "It's about time we had some tools to use, though I can't conceive of how intelligence sources could come up with the information before the lab. Even if we only have eighty doses, that's a start on finding out if it works. I'll get on the phone to the CDC and the manufacturer to scare up all we can get."

~

By seven a.m., Raines made the first notes of the improvement in most of the imipenem treated botulism patients. Within hours of receiving the new drug, their fever disappeared. Although their muscle weakness remained unchanged, it did not seem to progress to breathing difficulties. Most importantly, within two hours of receiving the miraculous intravenous antibiotic, the patients' diarrhea and cramping ended, reducing the risk of spreading the organism to others.

"Super!" replied Marshall after Raines gave him the preliminary results of the care begun on the advice of a spy. "I'll have the information on getting more of the drug by the time of the morning incident command meeting. Thanks—a lot."

Marshall hung up the phone, hopeful for the first time in three days. The Merck company executive he awakened volunteered all of the imipenem in stock on the factory's floor, and they promised shipment by air before nine a.m.

Chapter 46

EXECUTIVE POWER

Washington, D.C.; 19 September 2008

P resident Jack Lunsford started September 19th early, with phone calls to State and Defense, plus a private conversation with National Security Advisor George Tripp. At seven a.m., he entered the White House Situation Room, deep beneath the East Wing, to convene the emergency meeting of the National Security Council.

"Good morning, and be seated," directed the president. "I need your information and advice to formulate a response on the matter of foreign governmental involvement in the attack on Philadelphia."

"Mr. President," began FBI Director Chester Sheppard, "the recombinant DNA technology used in this attack originated in the Soviet Union and was imported to Iran by scientists who lost their jobs at *Biopreparat* at the end of the Soviet bioweapons program in 1992. The creation of this germ happened in an Islamic Republic laboratory facility financed by the Iranian government and with the oversight of an Iranian Intelligence officer. There is evidence that Iranian governmental rail and sea shipping assets were used to send this nightmare to our shores.

"There is no evidence to date that the French government was aware of the Logis Sourient shell company operating from France," Sheppard continued. "However, they have been less than candid with us on many previous occasions. The Norwegians ship thousands of containers daily and are only responsible for being unable to inspect them all. We have two of the individuals who carried out the Philadelphia attack and two of those apprehended in New York in custody, but they have given us little to no useful information. The creator of the germ, a Dr. Khalid Atoomb, has been more helpful. A clear chain of records exits that the Al-Douri Mosque's Delaware Bay Benevolence Fund funded the group. The remaining three perpetrators of the Philadelphia attack are deceased, as is one of the would-be New York attackers.

CIA Director Edward Rollins was next to brief the president.

"We have Dr. Atoomb in custody at Camp Peary. He is an Iraqi national working for the Iranian government, and universities in the United States trained him to be the creator of this deadly microorganism. He has been forthcoming with information on the production operation, his superiors, and even the antibiotics that are useful in stopping the infection. He seems to know nothing of the funding of the research on the germ.

Rollins thumped the table before him with his pen and continued.

"However, we have an excellent trail of large amounts of money that funded the American end of the operation. These funds include cash from the Brotherhood of Islamic

Jihad, the International Muslim Benevolence Fund, and the Muslim Liberation Front. These monies came into the Al-Douri Mosque and went directly into the Delaware Bay Benevolence Fund. We have arrested four of the leaders of the mosque, including the imam, as accessories to murder, and charged them with racketeering through the RICO Act. Secretary Hartford has more information on the organizations and our financial options."

Treasury Secretary John Hartford straightened in his chair and looked down at his notes.

"Mr. President," he began, "the Muslim Liberation Front and the International Benevolence Fund both have accounts associated with the Saudi Bukara Bank. Since the Bukara Bank has a branch office in New York, we in effect have the presence of these organizations on U.S. soil, and are able to freeze the assets of both of these organizations. The Brotherhood of Islamic Jihad will be a bit more difficult, since they bank through Damascus, but our legal people are actively investigating possible routes of attack."

"Good enough," said Lunsford. "The best way to stop such attacks is to destroy the organizations that fund them. Marilyn, what is the advice of State?"

"We feel strong economic actions are in order in respect to Iran, but not the threat of military action," began Secretary of State Marilyn Weinberg. "We suggest that we push for concessions to put the government in line with the actions of the rest of the planet. Iranian Ambassador Alwani is scheduled to arrive later this morning, as you have requested, but we have not briefed his office on the content of the planned discussions."

"Hugh," requested the president, "what are your recommendations?"

Secretary of Defense Hugh O'Conner was a lifetime soldier whose service dated back to the jungles of Vietnam and ended its uniformed phase as a major general in command of the

3rd Infantry Division. In the suit of the SECDEF, he spoke from the perspective of someone who understood the risks of placing men and women in harm's way. His responses were calm and measured.

"Sir, if your decision is a military approach, the joint chiefs would recommend a limited operation, launched from Iraq and Kuwait, with the objective of controlling Tehran and the 70 percent of the Iranian population that live there. The forces would primarily be light infantry of the 82nd and 101st Airborne divisions, air-assaulted into the capital to take down the government with the backup of the Air Force for laser-guided attacks on selected governmental targets. We would also advise precision munitions directed at the numerous chemical and biological facilities within a few hundred miles of the capital. The two nuclear development facilities pose more of a problem; since we are not sure how far along the Iranians are on their nuclear weapons production program. For these targets, we would advise surgical strikes with special operations troops to assess the full capacity of the plants before we destroy them. The operation would be expensive … and very unpopular in the Arab world."

"What is the earliest possible time frame for an action?" asked the president.

"Around sixty days," replied O'Conner, "since we have basing and air assets already in Iraq."

"How deeply are the Saudis involved?" Lunsford asked.

"A significant portion of the Philadelphia attack was funded through Saudi banks, but we do not have evidence of direct governmental support," replied Director Rollins.

"And the Syrians?"

"No evidence of official governmental knowledge," added Rollins.

With her words emphatic, Secretary Weinberg spoke up.

"Mr. President, State is very concerned that if we choose the military option, the U.S. position may well become untenable in the peace initiatives of Iraq and Palestine. There are three billion Muslims sharing our planet, and the backlash would likely be horrendous if we attack one of the two fully Islamic governments that now exist."

Chapter 47

BIG STICK

Washington, D.C.; 20 September 2008

Iranian Ambassador Ahmed Alwani sat uneasily in the Oval Office, awaiting the meeting requested by the most powerful man in the world. At 9:10 a.m., President Jack Lunsford entered the room, flanked by his chief of staff and national security advisor.

Alwani attempted to stand on shaky legs, but Lunsford waved him back into his chair and offered no words of greeting.

"Mr. Alwani," began the president, "your government has perpetrated an unprovoked attack on the citizens of the United States and we are here to discuss our options. Scientists housed and supported by the Islamic Republic have created a monster microorganism that threatens the safety of the world and is responsible for the deaths of more than two thousand of the people of Philadelphia and the illness of another two thousand."

A thin sheen of sweat became visible on Alwani's forehead as he stammered, "Mr. President, certain militant individuals within our government may have had knowledge of this terrible activity, but I assure you that the Islamic Republic holds no ill will toward the United States. I am quite sure that a formal apology will be forthcoming from my government."

"Mr. Alwani," continued the president grimly, "I have several thousand families in Pennsylvania who do not give a damn about your apology! The decision of whether or not to lay waste to your country is on the table. For you to avoid that fate will require changes in your government and your policies."

"What changes do you speak of?" asked the clearly shaken Alwani.

"The total cessation of work on nuclear armaments and restriction of your nuclear capacity to power production," began the president, "verified by United Nations Special Commission inspectors on a random-access basis. Secondly, the destruction of chemical and biological weapons within your borders, also verified by random inspection."

"It would be very difficult to persuade—" began Alwani.

The president interrupted him.

"It will be very easy for the United States to persuade the new government that will be in power in Iran," President Lunsford said. "The terms of the United States are not negotiable."

~

French Ambassador Francois Benoit sat aristocratically in the Oval Office, awaiting his conversation with President Lunsford. He was a frequent visitor to the White House, but usually for more pleasant reasons.

President Jack Lunsford entered the Oval Office with National Security Advisor George Tripp.

"Good morning, Mr. Ambassador," began a grim-faced Lunsford.

"Good morning, Mr. President," recited Benoit. "Thank you for your invitation to the Oval Office."

"I'm afraid the occasion is neither social nor pleasant, Mr. Benoit," Lunsford continued. "France has harbored the means for the shipment of weapons of terror into the United States. I need to know what your government knows of the situation and what you plan to do about it."

"I am very sorry for the loss of American lives, Mr. President, but France could not possibly have had any knowledge of such terrorists! We neither harbor militants nor encourage their presence in our country."

"I'm sure," replied Lunsford, briefly smiling before his countenance again turned cold. "Just as you had no knowledge of your Roland missiles that we found in Iraq in 2003 ... The bigger question is: what are you going to do about the fermenting of terrorists in your corner of Europe?"

"I'm not sure what measures—" Benoit began before being cut off by an angry Marine pilot.

"Mr. Benoit," Lunsford stated firmly, "I have on my desk an order for a U.S. embargo of *all* French imports, with particular emphasis on ending French wine sales in the United States within twenty-four hours. The order will also bar travel of all U.S. citizens into France without prior authorization of the State Department. Will you develop a plan with your government for the suppression of terrorism, or do I sign the order?"

"Mr. President," the pale Benoit replied, "be assured that France will undertake all possible initiatives to uncover and arrest those in France who are supporters of international terrorism. I give you my word and the word of the French government."

"Your word is more than adequate, Mr. Ambassador," smiled the president. "Thank you for coming."

~

The French ambassador hurriedly left the Oval Office, his worried facial features easily apparent to Christoffer Hallvard, the waiting Norwegian ambassador. As Hallvard entered the Oval Office, the president rose and offered a restrained greeting.

"Mr. President," began Hallvard intuitively, "we share a common problem in our shipping industries, in that there are too many containers, and containers are moved too quickly for the levels of security required for international safety. My government proposes a new system to ensure security, a 'reverse customs' process in which the exporting country is responsible for inspecting all rail, air, and sea shipping containers and providing an 'export seal' to ensure the safety of the importing country."

"That sounds like an excellent solution," said Lunsford. He added thoughtfully, "It will require additional customs personnel for all of us but will make the world a safer place. Could you be free tomorrow to explain your concepts to our Homeland Security and Customs departments?"

"Of course, Mr. President." smiled Hallvard with a sigh of relief.

President Jack Lunsford looked through the Oval Office windows, always enthralled by the peaceful appearance of the White House lawn, despite the immense pressures of the seat behind the *Resolute* desk.

"George," he pondered aloud to his chief of staff, "I'm going to give the Iranians forty-eight hours. Just forty-eight hours to do the right thing."

Chapter 48

NEW DAWN

Philadelphia; 20 September 2008

The Crisis Center had used the new intravenous imipenem therapy for a mere twenty-four hours before Marshall was able to release more than three hundred patients, beginning on September 20th. The ventilated and weakened patients were not yet showing muscular improvement, but the Crisis Center patients with diarrhea and fever began to improve after a single dose of the antibiotic. The Marine and National Guard microwave teams were rejoicing, and FEMA had announced that a cure was available that would stop the progression of the infection. People began to return to the streets of Philadelphia.

Dr. Ron Raines was enjoying his first quiet shift since the attack. Only two patients with diarrhea presented to the emergency department during the first hours of his shift, and with prompt imipenem therapy, their symptoms had resolved. He planned to register them as documented botulism patients, release them, and have them follow up at the Crisis Center at eight in the morning. The change in the disease's pattern was remarkable. Raines sat at the triage desk, charting patient improvements, when Christie approached.

"Ron," asked Christie Fellows, almost shyly, "got a minute to talk?"

"Yeah, sure," Raines answered.

"I know you've been through a lot over the last week, not only working so hard here, but losing Aimee," Christie said hesitantly. "I just wondered … how *you're* doing."

Raines considered the genuine concern voiced by the young nurse. Red-haired Christie, flamboyant and usually the first to joke, was now all serious business. It was a side of her he had not expected.

"Thanks for asking, Christie," he pondered, "but I don't think I even know the answer to that. I guess I've put myself so deeply into this mess that I haven't taken time to feel anything."

"Well, you're human too," she said.

"The funny thing is," Raines thought aloud, "I was once a doc with special operations troops, hell-bent on changing the world and being an instrument of national policy. When I decided that I should just live a peaceful life and take care of patients, I landed right in the middle of some serious international politics."

"I just wanted you to know I was worried about you," Christie smiled, revealing a small dimple at the right corner of her mouth. "How about breakfast on me?"

Raines thought about his job and his gratitude for the opportunities to move beyond his childhood. He thought about Tony Mateo and the fact that somewhere, he now had a grieving widow. Had there ever been anyone, other than his father, who really cared what was happening to him? It would be a new experience if he found that just acknowledging his fear of acceptance actually made it better. He had been a meal ticket and a step on the ladder for Aimee, but this young woman seemed to have different motivations ... although he really didn't understand why. He did not know if honest and kind people really existed ... but maybe they did.

"You know." Raines said, "sometimes life's changes are really for the better. I guess it's the 'Big Plan of Things.'"

Ron then nodded and said with enthusiasm, "Yeah ... breakfast together sounds really great."

Chapter 49

SOLITARY

Camp Peary, Virginia; 21 September 2008

In a solitary confinement cell in an unremarkable area of Camp Peary, Ahmed Madawi reviewed his options. He was deeply sorry that he had not thought quickly enough to fire on the American agents, for then it would all be over—the waiting all over and the martyrdom completed.

To die in Jihad would have been much better than this, he thought. To remain in the hands of these unbelievers for an untold number of years would be an unspeakable wrong.

Madawi sat cross-legged on the cell floor as his hands worked beneath the iron-framed bed. He carefully turned the toothbrush over and rubbed the left side of its handle against the concrete floor. It was not much of a weapon, but it was the only object available. He would be ready, and when the time presented itself, he would take an infidel with him to his grave.

Dr. Khalid Atoomb sat in a solitary cell less than fifty yards from the cells of the three Faithful. He did not know their names or that, if it were not for the soundproof door and walls, they would have been within range of his voice. It was frighteningly quiet and he did not know what would happen next. He had traded information only when he had no other choice, but he still had no knowledge of the Americans plans for his punishment.

Strangely, Atoomb felt, he had not enjoyed the satisfaction he had expected from the delivery of the Germ. No changes in the American ideology had yet occurred, and Madmudiyeh remained safe behind his guards in Tehran.

These walls are just as solid as they would have been in Iran if I had failed at my task, he lamented. The Faithful had dealt their blows to the infidels, but the secular government still stood—and perhaps now even grew stronger by the lessons it had learned.

I fear we have just fed the beast, and I will suffer its wrath for the rest of my days, he thought.

Atoomb's one remaining secret was the magazine mailing list. He would keep the information on the final blow deep inside until the illnesses started. They would then be desperate to know the source and would bargain with him.

As Atoomb sat on the cold, gray floor of the cell, he felt the beginning of a deep, cramping pain in his lower abdomen. Cold sweat appeared on his forehead as he realized the source of his peril.

How do I get imipenem in this hellhole?

Chapter 50

HOUSE CALL

Philadelphia; 21 September 2008

Dr. Ron Raines signed the last chart and rose to leave the department. Suddenly, he noticed a well-dressed man of sixty whose face he thought he should know. The man smiled and walked toward Raines, just as the doctor realized that the face was on a portrait he had seen in the doctor's lounge. It belonged to the hospital's administrator.

"May I speak to you, Dr. Raines?" asked Mr. Dubose. "I wanted to thank you for your excellent service to our hospital and the city during the botulism crisis," he said as he extended his hand.

"I guess I relearned a few things about not retiring from the responsibilities of being an American citizen," Raines smiled as he took the offered hand.

"But your assistance has been specifically requested

with another patient, Dr. Raines," Dubose added. "A White House figure asked this morning that we make you and Miss Fellows available to the government for a few days because of your experience in stopping the initial phases of the botulism infection. The officials asked that you prepare to treat a botulism-infected patient outside of the city and that you bring the medical supplies that you would need for controlling the active phase of the disease."

"Where are there other patients?" asked Raines.

"Sorry," shrugged Dubose, "I guess I'm not cleared to know that. The White House requested that the two of you prepare for a noon departure after meeting your transportation here in the emergency department. Thanks again for all you have done."

Raines wondered what type of high profile patient would be under the White House's scrutiny and how this person came to be exposed to the microorganism, and then he began to see the links to the recently provided antibiotic information. Whoever knew that the Enterobacter germ was sensitive to imipenem was in close proximity to its creation, and might even be the creator himself.

He placed the IV fluids and imipenem into a box for the trip and added meds for nausea and pain. He wished he still had his old army medic's aid bag to keep him company on the trip, but he thought that his White House–selected assistant just might make for more pleasant company than he remembered on army trips.

As Christie entered the nursing station, Raines noticed how tired she looked.

"What's this all about, Ron?" she asked.

"I'm not sure," he answered, "but if it interests the White House, I suspect we can guess how this high-profile patient was exposed to the germ. He or she may have been present at the creation end of this chain of horrors. I'm curious to see what kind of monster could be involved in such a plot."

Christie looked into the box and shook her head at the glaring holes she could see in the physician's preparations. She quietly began to gather her own list of needed items and smiled at the look of concentration on Raines's face.

At five minutes before noon, Raines looked up to see a familiar rumpled suit near the triage doors.

"Your taxi awaits, doc," said Talbot as his security-conscious gaze traversed the department and found no features of concern. Raines and Christie followed the intelligence agent through the doors, where they saw a blue-and-white Bell Jet Ranger on the helipad with rotors already turning. Talbot opened the rear cabin door and watched the medical professionals buckle in and place their boxes of supplies beneath the seat. The agent then took the copilot seat and gave the pair a "thumbs up" as the helicopter rose, dipped its nose, and followed its spinning rotor blades to the south.

After leaving Philadelphia's streets and Interstates, the helicopter ranged over patchy, rural Delaware forests with its shadow jerkily dancing among the treetops. Raines could see Washington in the west as the craft followed the expanse of the Chesapeake Bay southward, saw the islands at the bay's division, and could follow the Delmarva Peninsula and Cape Charles southward into Virginia.

After an hour and ten minutes of flight time, the chopper began to descend near a rural airstrip that Raines guessed to be in Virginia, just to the west of the Chesapeake. Nestled into the wooded setting he could see several new dormitories, a running track, and what he thought was a firing range. The Jet Ranger landed lightly on a concrete pad near a low profile, brown brick building that flew an American flag but was otherwise unmarked. As he followed Talbot and Christie into the building, Raines noted the features of a medical clinic, including small number of charts, a doctor's scale, and a single computer terminal. A young man seated at the receptionist's desk nodded but did not speak.

The stark brown tile walls of the infirmary's corridor were similar to the functional but plain walls of the hospital emergency departments that the physician and nurse knew so well. Talbot escorted the medical providers to a small nurse's station that was empty except for an armed guard wearing jeans and a lightweight jacket. The guard nodded toward a wire-reinforced glass door with a man visible on a cot inside.

"There is your patient ..." Talbot said and nodded to the figure. "His name is Dr. Khalid Atoomb, and he's a microbiologist."

With Raines's suspicions that his patient must be one of the creators of the germ weapon confirmed, he had no idea what he would say to the man who was responsible for the hundreds of deaths Raines had witnessed over the past ten days. He forced himself to enter the hospital room, reminding himself of his Hippocratic Oath to "first do no harm." Christie followed the physician into the treatment room as though she were providing care for any other needy patient in her emergency department.

"I'm Dr. Ron Raines," he said simply, "and we are here to help you."

The small man on the cot wore glasses and had a receding hairline. His face was flushed with fever, his eyes were sunken and dark from his lack of sleep, and he appeared to be in pain. His eyes however, did not radiate the evil that Raines expected, but reflected only his curiosity.

Christie knelt before the Iraqi and explained that she would begin an intravenous line to allow them to give him an antibiotic medication and botulism antitoxin. She expertly accessed the vein in Atoomb's left forearm and taped the catheter onto his warm, sweaty skin.

"Why do you help me?" asked Atoomb. "Do you preserve me for additional punishment?"

"We are helping you because you are a human being," answered Raines as he searched the scientist's face for the reasons behind the man's actions.

"But I am your enemy!" Atoomb protested.

"Only by your choice," said Raines quietly.

"You Americans want to suppress Islam and the entire Arab race," Atoomb lectured.

"I have no more interest in suppressing Islam than I have in persecuting traffic lights," said Raines with finality. He attached the imipenem in piggyback fashion to Atoomb's intravenous line and watched the miracle drug drip slowly into the saline solution flowing into the scientist's arm.

Atoomb felt the need to explain his actions, the faults of the American government and his goals of protecting his people and himself, but the absence of hatred in Raines's eyes confused him. This man was also a soldier for the things he believed and was doing the job that he felt was the right thing to do.

Could I have I been wrong about these people? wondered Atoomb.

Chapter 51

HEALING

Philadelphia; 21 September 2008

Gary Schell closed his carry on and sat down in the wheelchair piloted by a muscular young nursing assistant. The dark face and eyes of the orderly accentuated the large, blazingly white teeth so theatrically revealed by his comfortable smile.

Dr. Jill Case patted Schell on the back.

"Thanks for being here, Gary," she said. "I'm glad you were here to give us your experience."

"I think there are easier ways to miss my shifts," replied Gary with a skyward roll of the eyes.

"Have a nice flight. We'll see you back in Trenton," added Case, not at all convinced that the gray-haired paramedic should make another DMAT journey. They had been lucky this time and had avoiding losing a man who had risked his job and safety for the benefit of others.

The team would remain another week to ten days to see the patients graduate from the Crisis Center and return to their homes. Case knew she would never be the same physician and would never take lightly the safety of her teaching hospital in New Jersey.

~

"Hey, Dad," called Natalie Winslow into the kitchen, "I need to let you know about something."

Forrest Winslow closed the microwave door on the three frozen dinners and walked into the den, where Natalie was finishing her homework. At twelve, she was the new "woman of the house" following Karen's death.

"What's up, honey?" asked the gaunt man with dark circles below his eyes.

"Carrie's friend Bethany started her period yesterday. Carrie thought that it was gross, but I talked to her about growing up and the things starting to happen to her body. She has reproductive health in school this year, but not till after Christmas."

"Period?" asked the dazed father. "She's only nine!"

"That's old enough, Dad," Natalie informed him from her newfound cache of worldly experience.

~

FBI Special Agent Landrum looked over the shoulders of two of the rookie agents working the phones. Despite the fact that there were six newbies on the task for more than eight hours, he was terrified that they would contact someone too late.

"How many?" he asked the young agent wearing a Grateful Dead T-shirt beneath an FBI windbreaker. The young man looked over the mailing list provided by the publisher of *Healthy Life* magazine and the highlighted names that required a second call to inform them of the risks of the "Longevity Tea".

"Roughly two-thirds down," he breathed, unable to conceal his irritation with Landrum's repeated need for progress reports. "About six hundred to go."

⁓

Let me guess, the germ is sensitive to imipenem," smiled Dr. Al Marshall.

"Yes ... imipenem ... and aztreonam," said Dr. Stallings of the Pennsylvania State Lab with disappointment.

"We found out about the imipenem yesterday," replied Marshall, "but the information on another antibiotic that works will be very helpful. Thanks for the call, doctor."

Al Marshall could not sleep, despite the relative quiet of the curtained area at the rear of the Convention Center. He decided to send a few e-mails and check the news of the world outside of Philadelphia. He was tired of the road—tired of the travel to exotic places to put out fires for the CDC. He had investigated infectious events in fourteen U.S. states, plus Africa, Honduras, Panama and Iceland, but perhaps he had never been a dedicated husband and father.

He did not know if his job had contributed to his wife's development of "other interests," but he suspected it had. What hurt the most was that they were her decisions. She made the decision to invite her lover into their home while he was away, and it had been her decision to end the marriage. He guessed it really did not matter anymore, but the failure of the marriage just had not been within his control.

Most importantly, it was now painfully clear that he couldn't chance the same fate with his daughter. Al Marshall made his decision. He would take Emory up on their longstanding offer of a nice, geographically stable Professor of Infectious Disease job.

"... wanted you to know that I love you and miss you," he wrote to Jenny, "and think I may be home in a few days. I'm going to change some things in our lives, because I have been

away from you too much. You are important to me. Love,
Dad."

Al Marshall pushed "Send" and felt contented for the first
time in months.

Chapter 52

CHRISTMAS TREE

Philadelphia Harbor; 24 December 2008

"There!" exclaimed Christie. "It's perfect!"

Ron Raines had to admit, it really was perfect. It was just a silly little Christmas tree, all aluminum foil with red and green balls that seemed a bit too large for its vintage seventies appearance. He had to admit, however, that it brightened up the space.

They were in the cabin of Ron's "new boat," which was not a new boat at all. He was actually the third owner and had bought the Catalina 30 sailboat at a fire sale price. Of course, he knew the price was low because the boat needed paint ... and sails, and engine work ... and almost everything else. However, the hull was solid, and he needed an outlet for his off days and he needed goals for the future.

Raines now avoided watching the news, because he felt

powerless to change the bad news he heard. He could change the old boat. Working on the boat had become his new way of winding down after a grueling shift. Just a few hours of painting and polishing swept away some of the frustrations of the world's problems that just were not correctable.

Sitting behind the rusting helm of the boat made him feel like a kid playing sea captain—and the fact that some citizens of the world could choose to kill off thousands of the residents of a city because of their religious point of view became a little less painful. In adjusting the spring lines to position the boat perfectly at the dock, he felt in control of something, a comforting thought in a world that just could not be trusted. The idea of a quiet sail on Delaware Bay became his new carrot on a stick, and the dream was now of a day with a vivid blue sky, the boat heeled to starboard, and Christie laughing on the foredeck. It seemed more reasonable a goal than changing the world's political climate.

"To our first sailing adventure," Christie toasted as she held up her champagne glass for his contact.

"And to my first mate," added Ron, still fascinated that another human could be actually be interested in his future. They climbed the cabin stairs and sat under the boat's bimini top upon the faded lazarette seats.

"Why didn't you want to do the *Today Show* thing?" Christie asked. "You would've been great as a TV star."

"I just think the attack should have the right faces for the public's memory," Ron said quietly, "and I think those faces are those of Marshall, Mateo, Krause, and Case."

He paused.

"But I'm equally sure that the most of the real heroes will try to dodge the coverage."

"I'm sure that's true of Krause, though I guess both the CDC and the DMAT could use the positive press coverage," she said.

"The DMAT stayed away from their usual jobs for three

weeks, except for the guy who went home early," Raines commented.

"Somebody left early?" asked Christie.

"Yeah, but he had to have a heart attack to get away," the doctor grinned.

"Do you think Captain Mateo was infected with the Jihad organism?" asked Christie.

"We'll never know," Raines said, "but I really think he just had too many birthdays and ran out of heartbeats. He was still playing a young man's game, but he had long since paid his debt to his country. I had the chance to meet Mrs. Mateo when she came to Philadelphia to retrieve the captain's body. She is as gentle and strong as I would have imagined her to be. She lost her 'John Wayne,' and our nation lost a great leader."

"I'm going to miss Karen, too," Christie frowned. "She was such a big sister to all of us ... and the ER will never be the same without her."

"The last of the patients were off life support and out of the Crisis Center by mid-October," said Raines, "but I hear that a couple of them are filing suits for damages against the Muslim Liberation Front and the Saudi bank."

"They'll never get to the rich men that really fund the fundamentalists," said Christie. "Some middleman will take the fall, if anybody does."

"Yeah ... I don't think that real justice exists in our lifetime on this planet," Raines agreed.

"I read in the paper that Atoomb turned 'state's evidence'," Christie said. "He plans to testify against the Iranian general and Ahmadi from that Biolimit company. Apparently, he's willing to say in an international court that the germ he created was willfully used by the Philadelphia cell for murder, although he can't testify about any of the living cell members. I guess the prospect of a shot at paradise through the electric chair wasn't that appealing to him."

"He's obviously a bright guy," Ron said, "but I wonder if the prison system can even total up how long 2,000 life sentences would be."

"What do you think would've happened if he hadn't told you about the *Healthy Living* mailing list attack?" Christy asked.

"The disease would have cropped up in hundreds of locations, likely within a few days of people opening the tea," Raines replied, "and it could easily have spread from those cities throughout the nation. I'm not sure why he decided to tell me ... but as an enemy, I guess I must've been a surprise. I understand the FBI still hasn't been able to find everyone on the mailing list.

"I guess the Philadelphia cell members and the Al-Douri mosque leaders will be fried as the scapegoats for all the deaths," Raines went on, "when the true evil lies in the conception and planning of an attack like this. I think that Atoomb was just a frightened little man, taught to hate us and to expect religious persecution. The 'Faithful' were just pitifully idealistic and badly influenced. A lot of Muslims are getting more interested in weeding extremists out of the religion."

"At least there were changes in Iran from all of this," Christie said. "The United Nations' temporary ban on nuclear arms in the Middle East won't be popular in either Israel or the Arab world, but maybe it will give the planet a chance to exist a bit longer."

"Do you think the U.S. learned from all this, Ron?" Christie asked. "Is it all over?"

"The world's knowledge of new ways to put itself into danger isn't going to reverse itself," Raines said with resignation. "No, Christie ... I'm afraid it's just beginning."